THE BENEFITS
OF MARIJUANA
Physical, Psychological
and Spiritual

by
Joan Bello

LIFESERVICES PRESS
Boca Raton, Florida

THE BENEFITS OF MARIJUANA
Physical, Psychological
and Spiritual

Published by LIFESERVICES PRESS
POST OFFICE BOX 4314
BOCA RATON, FLORIDA 33429
Email: tiffywiff2@aol.com
Revised Edition
Library of Congress Catalogue Card Number: 97-92699
ISBN 0-9660988-0-3
Printed in the U.S.A.

Acknowledgments

Invaluable contributions to this work were made by my loving husband, Andrew Bello, who spent many long evenings with me as we labored over this book to complete it. His relentless support, constant encouragement, and many suggestions gave us both the strength to continue during the most difficult time of our lives.

The conscientious expertise and patience of Barbra Haynes in preparing this manuscript cannot be measured, except to say that her effort was surely beyond the call of duty, even for a daughter.

Special thanks to Steve Willis for the front cover which portrays what this book needs 800,000 words to say.

And I am indebted to Jon Hanna (Soma Graphics) who volunteered his talent and focused attention to fine tune the manuscript and correct all the errors.

Don Wirtshafter (Ohio Hempery) offered his valuable knowledge, without being asked, solely to make this book as good as it could be.

James Dawson, a medical marijuana beneficiary and new but lifelong friend, afforded access to invaluable internet information with no motive except to help. We are all indebted to him.

And special appreciation must be extended to Michael Long, who spent countless hours researching for the revisions in this edition and without whose keen energy, committment, and support this printing would not have been possible.

I will always be grateful to Guy Mount (Sweetlight Books) who lent his inspiration and brilliance to Benefits.

Finally, I need to thank my father, Francis N. Sorrentina, who supported my work wholeheartedly even before he understood its righteousness. He has been the most alert, gentle, and steadfast influence of my entire life, for which I am eternally grateful.

The ultimate inspiration for this work, however, along with the intuitive understanding as to how and why to proceed is without question due to the guidance granted me by the mind and heart expansion of the marijuana plant.

❦

TABLE OF CONTENTS

LIFESERVICES
Box 4314 • Boca Raton, FL • 33429
(561) 750 - 0554
Email: tiffywiff2@aol.com

In these difficult social times, when the forces of ignorance
are encroaching upon the light, if truth and love are to have an arena of
possibility, the enlightened should join together.

With the growing evidence of the absolute wonder of marijuana as medicine, the government stands firmly against compassion and justice. While those in power are mocking the truth and calling it "the wrong message to the children," those in need are beginning to realize that tyranny must be countered with solidarity.

The ploy of using "the welfare of the children" in its sordid campaign against the truth carries with it the burden of neglect of countless numbers of sick people, a small sampling of whose need is documented in Appendix I.

WHEREAS:
• When the New England Journal of Medicine acknowledged the medical value of Cannabis
• Voters in California and Arizona supported medical marijuana
• National Institute of Health recognized the medical efficacy of Cannabis
• Initiatives in Washington and District of Columbia appear positive for medical marijuana

YET:
The Government of the United States continues to call the truth "wrong."

The Grassroots Association for Medical Marijuana (GRAMM) is a voice against the tyranny that is interfering with the freedoms of the choices of sick Americans.

The information on the following pages is offered to support the goal of allowing marijuana its rightful position in medicine.
If you use marijuana for a sense of general well-being, or if you believe that marijuana should be available to responsible adults as medicine, you can contact GRAMM at Lifeservices.

— Joan Bello
Lifeservices Press
September 26, 1997

PREFACE: A Letter From Jail
Dale R. Gowin

*Children of a future age
Reading this indignant page,
Know that in a former time
Love! sweet Love! was thought a crime.*
— *William Blake*

It is a great honor and privilege to introduce to the world Joan Bello's courageous and insightful treatise on the Benefits of Marijuana. Grounded in multidisciplinary science and bolstered by a wealth of documentation, this groundbreaking work provides ample evidence to support the intuitive knowledge of millions, that Cannabis offers healing potentials for the human body, mind, and spirit.

For too long, the many millions who have known this truth have cowered in fear beneath the shadows of deception and repression. In our own lives we have borne witness to the healing virtues and spiritual gifts bestowed by Nature through this plant, yet we have languished timidly as our liberty to pursue this happiness was stripped away; and we have watched in silence as our sisters and brothers were hauled away, their homes and property seized, for no crime other than peacefully partaking of, and sharing, the spirit-nurturing Light that is crystallized within the cells of this verdant and virtuous vegetable. No longer can we abide in this conspiracy of silence. The clarion call of Truth rings from these pages. An answering echo is the ancient promise of prophecy: The truth will set you free.

My relationship with cannabis began in 1967, when I was 17 years old. I discovered, to my amazement and delight, that this humble plant had the power to bestow the gift of Divine Grace to one who would respectfully partake of its resinous flowers and leaves. Its subtle magic gently lifted me from the doldrums of daily life, into realms of deeply enriched clarity of mind and vibrancy of vision. I gradually came to realize that the miraculous gift of consciousness enhancement granted by cannabis and the other psychedelic plants was the most valid, genuine, and authentic manifestation of Spiritual Light that I had ever encountered. Now, after 30 years largely devoted to the Spiritual Quest, this realization remains undimmed.

Ten years after first partaking of the Holy Herb, I crossed the Rubicon of personal commitment and devoted myself to public activism against prohibition. This inevitably led to my arrest in a "sting operation" and a 12-year prison sentence.

My research about the Holy Herb led to some truly amazing discoveries. Among the things I learned were these:

Cannabis (marijuana) was probably the first plant ever cultivated by humans. In the Neolithic period, as the glaciers of the Pleistocene ice age were receding from Earth's temperate zones, nomadic food gatherers collected Cannabis along with other wild plants. Its fertile seeds, a protein-rich food source, sprouted readily and grew abundantly in the disturbed soil near their campsites. The prevalence of the plant near Neolithic campsites and its ease of cultivation spurred the transition from a nomadic food-gathering economy to settled agriculture - a quantum leap in the evolution of human civilization.

Cannabis was a uniquely useful survival resource to our prehistoric ancestors. Every part of the plant had important uses. Fibers stripped from the stalks were twisted into twine for bows, fishing lines and snares, and were woven into fabric for clothing and canvas for shelter. The wood-like "hurds" inside the stalks were used as cooking and heating fuel. The seed, as well as providing sustaining food, was pressed for oil, providing light in our earliest earthenware lamps and pushing back the threatening shadows of night. The leaves and flowers were used as medicine - Cannabis is mentioned in the earliest extant herbals - and were used by shamans and worshipers as aids to spiritual revelation.

In more recent eras, the Cannabis plant was used extensively in industry for the manufacture of paper, plastics, fabrics, fuels, chemicals, cosmetics, and literally thousands of other products. It was the economic value of these applications - and its competitive threat to the monopoly profits of petroleum-based corporate cartels - that led to the imposition of Cannabis prohibition in the 20th century.

Cannabis was widely respected as a medicine since ancient times throughout the world. Before prohibition, the U.S. Pharmacopoeia listed over 100 approved uses for it, and it was one of America's most popular over-the-counter medications in the 19th century. Cannabis was the standard treatment for asthma, emphysema, epilepsy, migraine, arthritis, glaucoma, insomnia, and many other conditions. Recent research has shown that Cannabis is a safer and more effective treatment for many of these conditions than the expensive synthetic pharmaceuticals preferred by the monopoly-based medical establishment.

Cannabis has been recognized as a spiritual sacrament by virtually every religious tradition in the world. Chinese Taoists, Hindus from India, Tibetan Buddhists, the Gnostics and Essenes of Judaism, Coptic Christianity, the Sufi and Ishmaili traditions of Islam - all of these and more have known and respected the holiness and religious value of the Cannabis experience.

There is no truth to the government-sponsored propaganda about the alleged dangers of marijuana. From the "reefer madness" campaign of the 1930s to the claims made by DARE and the Partnership for a Drug Free America today, the prohibitionist rhetoric is nothing more than a smokescreen of lies and fabrications, promulgated by the Corporate-Monopoly State for economic and political purposes. Every unbiased scientific study has found that Cannabis is non-addictive, non-toxic, and potentially beneficial.

Joan Bello's illuminating text acknowledges the truth about Cannabis without kowtowing to the sacred cows of prohibitionist political correctness, and pushes the debate past conventional limits, into virgin territory fraught with relevance to today's most urgent social issues. A work of 21st-century science, this book sets the agenda for a new generation of discourse. The bold thesis presented in these pages is that Cannabis is not only harmless and benign as a recreational euphoriant, but also a holistic medicine for deep healing of the human body, mind, and spirit – and a specific remedy for the spiritual malaise of Western Civilization, the disastrous disharmony that characterizes this last decade of the Old Millennium. Cannabis played a vital role in human evolution thousands of years ago, providing sustenance and solace to the scattered survivors of the great glaciers. It may yet prove to be an equally important asset in our next great evolutionary hurdle as the human race faces the challenge of survival into the New Millennium.

As this book makes clear, Cannabis is an essential part of the natural birthright of all Earthdwellers, and its prohibition is truly a crime against humanity.

Dale R. Gowin, #91-B-0209
Midstate Correctional Facility
Marcy, New York

July 4, 1996

ORGANIZATIONS THAT HAVE ENDORSED MEDICAL ACCESS TO MARIJUANA INCLUDE:

- American Bar Association;
- American Medical Student Association;
- American Public Health Association;
- California Nurses Association;
- California Senior Legislature;
- Colorado Nurses Association;
- Congress of California Seniors;
- Federation of American Scientists;
- Lymphoma Foundation of America;
- National Association of Attorneys General;
- National Association of Criminal Defense Lawyers;
- National Nurses Society on Addictions;
- New York Nurses Association;
- Physicians Association for AIDS Care;
- Virginia Nurses Association;
- American Academy of Family Physicians;
- Burlington (VT) Board of Health;
- Mississippi Nurses Association;
- New Mexico Nurses Association;
- Northern New England Psychiatric Society;
- Virginia Nurses Society on Addictions;
- National Lymphoma Foundation;
- California Pacific Conference of the Methodist Church;
- Conference of Episcopal Bishops;
- National Association of People with AIDS;
- Florida Governor's Red Ribbon Panel on AIDS;
- Mothers Against Misuse and Abuse;
- Iowa - Civil Liberties Union, Democratic Party
- Minnesota Democratic Farm-Labor Party

EDITORIAL BOARDS THAT HAVE ENDORSED MEDICAL ACCESS TO MARIJUANA INCLUDE:

Boston Globe; Chicago Tribune; Miami Herald; New York Times; Orange County Register; USA Today.

Introduction

This book has gone through many printings since 1991. Originally, The *Benefits of Marijuana* was begun as a personal research project because I wanted to understand the process by which this plant enhanced my consciousness. There was no problem in discovering the historical utilizations of hemp/marijuana for fuel, fiber, food, medicine and even religious sacrament. I found numerous philosophical essays exalting "marijuana consciousness." But nowhere could I find a satisfactory discussion that explained by what physical mechanism the Cannabis Sativa plant gave extra depth to my perceptions. And, although I discovered references to specific maladies for which cannabis, in years past, was said to offer relief, no definitive scientific reason for its healing ability seemed to exist. While tests that proved its complete safety were in abundance, and ancient tomes spoke of it as a sacred "gift from the gods," in the modern literature, cannabis was portrayed as a very dangerous drug. It all added up to a mystery I needed to solve.

Meanwhile, national awareness concerning the issue of cannabis as medicine barely existed. The criminalization of recreational marijuana vs. the right of adults to choose their own vice was the popular controversy. Although many sick people were employing cannabis to relieve their symptoms, they were isolated from each other and silent about their need, purchasing pot on the black market when it was available and affordable. Some patients chose to grow their own, and many of these patients were arrested and imprisoned.

In the 70s and 80s thousands (perhaps millions) of seriously sick people did not have any idea that marijuana could lend comfort to their disease, and possibly offer a turning toward healing, if not physically, at least by unhinging them from the mental stress that exacerbates so many illnesses. Even many of the patients who enjoyed cannabis regularly, to feel and function better, harbored guilt over their use. Their personal experience contradicted everything they had been taught to believe. They were confused and did not understand how such a maligned substance could so enhance their well-being. I wrote this book because, after years of documented research, and through personal experience and formal training, I had come to understand the astonishingly simple mechanism by which marijuana benefits the physical, psychological and, in some cases, even the spiritual elements of human life. I was committed to sharing that knowledge.

Since I first started working on this project, there have been great strides in the hemp/marijuana movement. In the early nineties, a synchronous realization throughout the world of marijuana consciousness emerged concerning the benefits that this plant offers, and the importance of making this information available to the public. This realization grew to a crescendo (among people, who were otherwise completely unconnected) in response to any number of conjuncting factors. One of the earliest visible influences was Jack Herer's exposé, *The Emperor Wears No Clothes*, documenting that hemp has an almost unbounded potential for replacing environmentally-devastating industries. We can stop cutting forests down for paper, and instead grow hemp - without pesticides and without fertilizers. We can stop burning fossil fuels which poison our atmosphere, and instead grow hemp for biodegradable fuel. We can replace cotton, which entails using poisonous fertilizers and pesticides, we don't need synthetics manufactured from petrochemicals - we can just grow hemp. Neither do we need any petrochemicals for paints, or lumber from trees for building boards - all were shown as perfectly feasible utilizations of Hemp in Herer's revolutionizing work. As word spread, lists of specific diseases that could be medicated with cannabis - which actually had been medicated with cannabis for thousands of years - became well-known. Medicine that comforts, aids, strengthens and clarifies is the history and the potential of this outlawed plant. The situation for so many patients, once they were exposed to Herer's information, became one in which they realized that they were, first of all, not alone, and secondly, not mistaken concerning their personal experience. Their intuition was validated. Hemp / Cannabis / Marijuana made them feel good because it has very individual and measurable remedial effects for a number of diverse health problems.

With the birth of the internet, the hemp/marijuana patients and advocates were no longer isolated or in the dark. The information on Cannabis Sativa was limitless. There is no question that the technological wonder tool of the internet has made all the difference. With both knowledge and unity the move toward demanding recognition for marijuana as medicine has been energized.

And of course, Dr. Grinspoon , the Harvard doctor who has been an advocate for marijuana, since he first started his studies on the plant, back in the 70's has published moving testimonials from patients that have made a deep impact in the conventional field of medicine. Due largely to the efforts of Dr. Grinspoon, the *New England Journal of Medicine* expressed its support for medical marijuana. (January 30, 1997 - from Jerome P. Kassirer, M.D. - "I believe that a federal policy that prohibits physicians from alleviating suffering by prescribing marijuana for seriously ill patients is misguided, heavy-handed, and inhumane. Some physicians will have the courage to challenge the continued proscription of marijuana for the sick. Eventually, their actions will force the courts to adjudicate between the rights of those at death's door and the absolute power of bureaucrats whose decisions are based more on reflexive ideology and political correctness than on compassion.")

Dr. Grinspoon's latest book, *Marihuana: The Forbidden Medicine*, gives in-depth testimony from patients for whom cannabis represented their only effective and safe medicine. Over the years, his stance has become more bold, until he finally called marijuana - "the wonder drug of the century."

In the 80s, the U.S. government itself, recognized the need for cannabis therapeutics when it initiated the "Compassionate Protocol" for patients whose diseases responded only to cannabis. This was a well-kept secret and in 1992 as word leaked out and hundreds of AIDs patients signed up to be considered, the government closed the program. As we go to press, it still supplies 8 patients from the "compassionate program" with Mississippi-grown government cannabis (300 marijuana cigarettes a month are delivered to each of these patients).

While forces to illuminate the public as to the boundless medical applications of cannabis were growing exponentially, formidable resistance was building on the other side. We can never discount the fear that the marijuana mindset portends for a competitive-driven society. Marijuana is known to alter focus from a materialistic ethic to one of compassion and timeless values. It enhances tolerance and cooperation in direct opposition to the militaristic mentality of acquisition and domination, and consequently is a direct threat to the economic system and political establishment.

Despite the fact that the War on Drugs' mentality is constantly being fed a one-sided diet of fear from the authorities, in 1996 the voters in California and Arizona perceived what the truth actually is about cannabis as medicine and responded to the need of suffering patients, by sending the "right message" to the government. With passage of the grass-roots-driven Initiative, known as Proposition 215 (The Compassionate Use Proposition), doctors in California were given the right to prescribe cannabis for severe discomforts and diseases. In Arizona, Proposition 200 allows doctors to prescribe cannabis, as well as to introduce other controlled substances into treatment plans, when appropriate

Doctors considering recommending medical marijuana, to patients, even though in line with state law as authorized by a direct vote of the people, were warned that Federal prosecution could follow any such suggestion. ("U.S. Government to Prosecute Doctors who Prescribe Marijuana" - *N.Y. Times,* 12/23/96) As a result of this threat, doctors-in-good standing filed a Federal lawsuit questioning the constitutionality of such an intrusion into patient/doctor confidentiality. Meanwhile the government agencies continue to ignore all the scientific studies that clearly show marijuana's unique and magnificent efficacy in easing the pain and suffering of numerous ailments.

In 1944, Mayor LaGuardia's Committee on Marijuana completely discredited all of the reasons for outlawing hemp/marijuana in the first place. After specifically testing whether or not marijuana represented any health hazard whatsoever to the community, the committee categorically stated that it did not, either by way of deleterious effects to the body or the mind of the user, or even to the community at large. It further attested to the non-addictiveness of marijuana use and to its therapeutic possibilities:

> The lessening of inhibitions and repressions, the euphoric state, the feeling of adequacy, the freer expression of thoughts and ideas, and the increase in appetite for food, brought about by marijuana suggests therapeutic possibilities. (Summary by George B. Wallace, Chairman)

In 1988, Court Hearings were held to determine whether or not marijuana had any medicinal value. The DEA's own Law Judge,

Francis Young gave his decree after studying the evidence over a two year period:

> By any measure of rational analysis, marijuana can be safely used within a supervised routine of medical care....and marijuana is one of the safest therapeutically active substances known to man!

Again, the truth is ignored. The DEA Administration maintains the "Schedule I" status for marijuana: "Dangerous, with no medical value." That categorization was again challenged in the courts in 1994. Again all the evidence as to its safety, medical uses, and current medical documentation was ignored, strongly suggesting that the facts about cannabis have nothing to do with its prohibition.

The right to use marijuana as a personal choice has found acceptance with governments throughout the world, but these widescale global changes in international marijuana law have hardly been reported here in the U.S. Our media is guilty of selective journalism, and in the wake of recent international changes, our government is guilty of ostrich-like behavior.

In Columbia, South America, owing to the universal recreational acceptance of marijuana, it became legal to possess up to one ounce for personal pleasure. On the other side of the earth, in Germany, Switzerland, and the Netherlands, almost in time sync with the Colombian about-face, it became legal to posses up to one ounce. The Netherlands has further extended that license to include distributing marijuana – up to one ounce – through the mail. Motivation for these major changes in so many industrialized nations came about through the explosive populations of minor drug-charged inmates in the prison system. The financial drain of their fragile economics proved to be of more importance than the disfavor of the American government. Although that disenchantment with Columbia's court-sanctioned easing of the marijuana laws was loud and acerbic, hardly any mention of any of these happenings was reported by or to the mainstream. The world is likewise embracing the hemp/marijuana plant for its many varied uses in industry. Hemp is actually becoming a major crop once again – in all but America.

Switzerland and Holland both grow and distribute "medical grade" hemp. Doctors in those countries are doing testing for understanding the specific reasons that marijuana is so beneficial for so many diseases. The latest suggestion for sanity comes from France's Environment Minister Dominique Voynet: "As a politician and a trained medical doctor, I favor legalizing cannabis. While heroin addiction often affects people predisposed to drug addiction, the occasional consumption of cannabis has no effect on health and social relations." (Sept. 17, 1997, Reuter) With National Institute of Health acknowledgment of the medical potentials of cannabis (1996), it is hoped that similar tests will be conducted in the U.S. although no plans have yet been finalized or even sanctioned.

If the end results of this long-standing campaign against such a magnificent plant were not completely destructive for the earth and fraught with pain, suffering, and anguish for so many people, we could almost laugh at the silliness of it all. Here is a plant that grows with the utmost of ease, everywhere. Here is the Hemp plant that can underwrite the commercial needs of the entire global economy, without pesticides / fertilizers / mega machines, and without any devastation to the atmosphere or the life forms of the planet. Here is Cannabis Sativa, which was always a medicine for as far back as humans kept records (and before that). It helps every instability of the human organism. Ancient and modern studies have demonstrated its value and its safety. More in-depth studies have been conducted on the marijuana plant than on any other.

The government sanctions a synthetic pill (Marinol) for medicine which mimics the active ingredient in the hemp flower for medical purposes. This "Marinol" pill has side effects and warnings of overdose. Nevertheless, during studies conducted in California from 1981 - 1989 (California Research Advisory Council) measuring the effectiveness for nausea either of Marinol or the natural herb, children in the study had to be over 15 years of age if they were in the controlled part of the study using the natural ingredients. To use the synthetic, however, children as young as 5 were accepted into the study. (Results were statistically significantly in favor of the natural herbal)

The U.S. government supplies 8 persons with marijuana for medical conditions - every month. Voters in two states, Legislatures in 34 states, Courts in 3 states, and the domain of the District of Columbia - all have acknowledged the medical efficacy of marijuana. Doctors and their patients are suing the government to have the right to follow the vote of the majority (in California and

Arizona) and be allowed to prescribe the best and safest medicine for every condition.

In the first analysis, the opposition to utilizing marijuana for its myriad purposes seems to be the government. On closer observation it is easy to see that the industries who would lose power if the infinite possibilities of marijuana are unleashed are really the power behind prohibition. Not just logging companies, or oil giants, not just cotton farmers/manufacturers, not only pharmaceutical companies. Freedom for cannabis represents great loss to the booming prison/legal industry. Despite all the underhanded tactics to discredit marijuana, and to maintain prohibition, regardless of the cost to taxpayers or the suffering of patients or the anguish of families destroyed by the penal system, patients and advocates for cannabis and for freedom, continue to push forward. 1997 will be witness to more Voter Initiatives. By all polling sophistication, it appears that the District of Columbia and the state of Washington will have voter-passed state laws that allow their seriously ill citizens access to Cannabis Therapeutics. 1998 will see even more states take the vote directly to the people. From the time I first began my work on *Benefits of Marijuana*, it seems we have really progressed.

For me, this last year has served as my greatest progression in understanding the wonders of marijuana. Up until now (1997), this book represented technical study, including all kinds of academic research. It was framed under my own holistic orientation taking into account observations of many years, as well as self-study.

However, in no way was I prepared for what I learned first-hand, from the patients. Nothing I read or wrote was as shocking as the absolute savior-like effects of marijuana on the hundreds of seriously ill patients whom I was honored to interview while working as an Intake Counselor for the law offices of Lawrence Elliott Hirsch.

When I first put forth the hypothesis that cannabis balanced the Autonomic Nervous System, out from which all kinds of health benefits can develop - there were no people to validate this reasoning. With the publication of the revised edition of *Benefits of Marijuana,* I have been able to include only some of the patients and just the briefest summary of their need and the relief that cannabis affords. APPENDIX I (Patient Testimonials) shows - beyond a shadow of a doubt, that marijuana is indeed a "wonder medicine."

The Action Class For Therapeutic Cannabis was developed by Larry Hirsch and Hirsch & Caplan Public Interest Law Firm in Philadelphia, Pennsylvania.

"I am extremely gratified in the progress that we have made in putting together what we feel is one of the most important cases in the history of the United States. Plaintiff-class representatives now number more than two hundred and come from every state in the union. They share the common issue of being candidates for the free and legal use of therapeutic cannabis for their health, wellness, and quality of life. The class action is in its final stages of preparation and will be filed in the near future.

This has been an enormous undertaking that has been carried entirely by Hirsch & Caplan Public Interest Law Firm. Special thanks go to Michael Long, Ryan Perlman, Carol Kaplan, James Dawson, Kay Lee and Joan Bello, whose dedication and hard work have been essential to our progress."

Peace, Love and Victory For the People"

Lawrence Elliott Hirsch
Hirsch & Caplan Public Interest Law Firm
1700 Sansom Street, Suite 501
Philadelphia, PA 19103
Toll Free:
1-888-LEH-LAW1
1-888-LAW-WAR1
Fax:
215-496-9532
E-Mail:
LEH36@aol.com
lehlaw@netreach.net

Chapter 1 • The Effect of Marijuana
Classification of Marijuana

It is little wonder that the unique makeup of marijuana has caused major confusion over its effects on the human body. Neither a stimulant nor a depressant, pharmacologically it is classified by itself (Weil, 1980, Chapter 10; Schultes and Hofmann, 1979, p. 93). That it produces changes in mood has allowed for its classification as a hallucinogen, but this definition is ultimately unsatisfactory, since hallucinogens are chemically unrelated to the molecular makeup of marijuana. Plant hallucinogens and hormones manufactured in the brain are both water soluble: They both contain nitrogen and are categorized therefore as alkaloids. But the marijuana compound has no nitrogen, and its active principles occur in a resinous oil; they are not released in water.

> Almost all plants that alter consciousness contain the element nitrogen and therefore belong to the large class of chemical compounds known as alkaloids. Among the more important plants with psychoactive properties, only Hemp (marijuana) has active principles which do not contain nitrogen. (Shultes and Hofmann, 1979, p. 172)

The alteration in mental processes that takes place with hallucinogens occurs because of their similarity to brain hormones. The usual pathways of neuronal messages within the brain change dramatically and directly when hallucinogens are introduced. But marijuana does not affect this mechanism at all. Instead its effects on brain patterns are indirect and are mediated through the more subtle regulation of the autonomic nervous system (ANS), as will be explained in the following pages.

To classify marijuana as a drug ignores both its physiological effects and its chemical makeup. The term "drug" connotes concentration of a substance to its most powerful form, but marijuana is unprocessed, dried vegetation from a strong smelling annual herb called cannabis. It maintains its natural complex chemistry of both active and inactive compounds rather than concentration of a single compound.

> The relationships people form with plants are different from those they form with white powders...users tend to stay in better relationships with them over time. One reason for this difference

is that plants are dilute preparations, since the active principles are combined...with inert vegetable matter...Doctors and pharmacologists refer to these predominating chemicals as the active principles of the plants, which would be fine except that it implies all the other constituents are inactive and unimportant. (Weil and Rosen, 1983, p. 31)

The main problem with drugs is their danger, since all drugs are defined as poisonous, depending upon dose, which means overdose can cause death. However, marijuana has no known level of toxicity. The amount needed to produce a lethal reaction has been estimated at from eating five pounds at one time, to smoking 40,000 joints in one day, far beyond any physical possibility (NORML, 1995). "It does not kill people in overdose or produce other symptoms of obvious toxicity." (ibid.)

The term "narcotic" describes a drug or poison that reduces sensibility by depressing brain function, which can cause death by stopping respiration. Because marijuana has none of these effects, its legal classification as a narcotic is completely without basis. "Guided by the...(Victorian) ethic, the U.S...easily made the mistake of classifying marijuana as a narcotic: in point of fact, it is a mild euphoriant." *(Editor's note in the 1973 re-publication of Mayor's Committee, NYC, 1944, piii.)*

Since marijuana contains at least 421 complex molecules (NORML 1995; Howlett et. al., 1990; Herer 1985, p. 32; Cohen, 1975), all attempts to understand how it works by the usual modern method of isolating each part and testing its effects have failed. Because of these failures, many grave misconceptions have developed, "its effects are hard to describe because they are so variable" (Weil and Rosen, 1983, p.115).

Scientific and Scholarly Studies

Over the last century, published scientific investigations conducted by the governments of India, Costa Rica, Jamaica, Greece, Canada, the U.S. and the city of New York have all concluded that marijuana is not only the safest recreationally used substance, but also has unmistakably unique therapeutic properties. Since the 1960s marijuana has been the subject of thousands of studies by the U.S. Government, pharmaceutical companies, and private agencies. Even though the investigations funded by the U.S. Government and pharmaceutical companies set out specifically to prove the harmfulness of marijuana, the evidence was quite the contrary. Time and again untested and preposterous allegations have been highlighted in the press, such as, that marijuana caused birth defects, brain damage, lung cancer, and sterility. However, these accusations have been scrutinized and proven untrue. The last government-sponsored investigation began in the Nixon years and was finally completed during Carter's term. Marijuana was almost decriminalized at that time because the Commission could find no danger whatsoever issuing from its use, either for health or behavior, but because of fierce political pressures from the hard-core conservative elements, marijuana remained stigmatized and illegal.

It should be noted that in the Spring of 1996, the American Medical Association (AMA) was about to publicly declare itself in favor of legalizing marijuana at one of its symposiums, but this was nipped in the bud in the nick of time by the politicized right (N.Y. Times, *AMA Shelves,* 1996). This action was nearly taken because of the increasing number of therapeutic benefits for which marijuana can no longer be ignored: AIDS-related symptoms, chemotherapy-caused nausea, glaucoma, asthma, spasticity, phantom pain, emphysema, epilepsy, stress, and loss of appetite. The extent of these therapies (for which marijuana's benefits are well-known) points unmistakably to a dramatic healing effect on the entire organism. But still no one can believe the obvious. Many of the private studies (before the ban on marijuana research in '72) presented a wealth of information, indicating possible medical and psychiatric applications, but their findings were not integrated into a general holistic understanding. Since that time the only studies exempted from this ban were undertaken by pharmaceutical companies with the sole intention of manufacturing synthetic compounds which can be patented.

To be fully understood, marijuana's effects must be viewed holistically. The complexity of action of the 421+ known chemicals cannot be divided and then explained as the product of the total response. While one cannabinoid compound acts in one direction, yet another moderates the first, and so on down the line, perhaps 421 times. Only complete consideration of the innumerable elements (both active and inactive) will serve up the reality of their total effect. And only by observation of the total reaction within the body and on the person can we begin to clear up the confusion about the effect of cannabis on the human body. To understand this action, we need to understand the Autonomic Nervous System.

Autonomic Nervous System

The Autonomic Nervous System (ANS) might well be called the Eighth Wonder of the World. Our heart beat, our breath, our temperature, our appetites, all our cellular exchanges are regulated by this automatic pilot. It sends the right signal, to the right organ, at the right time – without conscious knowledge or effort. The primary control center is the hypothalamus (section of the brain) which activates automatic processes in accordance with the body's needs at any moment.

Marijuana (comprising various cannabinoid compounds) molecules fit "pharmacologically distinct receptors" within this complicated mechanism.

> The key to understanding how the brain communicates through this array of chemical messages lies in the shape of the chemicals and their receptors. Distributed throughout the body on the surface of cell membranes are hundreds, perhaps thousands of different types of molecular structures called receptors. Each type of receptor has a characteristic 3-dimensional shape and, like a lock, can only be opened or activated by a chemical key with the correct corresponding shape. (Ornstein/Sobel, 1990, p. 88-89) Howlett (1989): "This cellular selectivity provides evidence for the existence of specific receptors for the cannobimemetic...The hypothesis can be proposed for a 'cannabinoid' receptor...and findings suggest...a pharmacologically distinct receptor."

This "fit" has led to much speculation in the scientific community concerning the ancient evolutionary connection between the marijuana plant and human ancestry.

Scientists have just discovered that there is a brain hormone that is keyed to this receptor (Devane, 1994; Mechoulam, 1990). Preliminary testing has demonstrated its identical effects with the THC molecule. This "new" brain chemical (which unlocks the same receptor as the THC molecule) clarifies that the effects of the cannabinoids are completely compatible to our organisms. Our own brain produces "Anandamide," appropriately named after the Indian word for "bliss." What is truly amazing is that the natural brain chemical is a completely different shape than the cannabinoid molecule, suggesting a subtle, electromagnetic twin charge between the plant compound and the brain hormone, not yet detectable.

The ANS operates through two branches, the Sympathetic and the Parasympathetic, each exerting its opposing influence in constant complex chemical cooperation to balance the body (homeostasis) under all conditions. The ANS is made up of chains of two kinds of neurons that travel from the brain and spinal column to organs throughout the body. Increasing Sympathetic activity results in outpourings of the body's chemical stimulants, whereas additional Parasympathetic action is accommodated by the body's chemical depressants.

The ANS is intimately connected to the mind so that when we interpret our situation as safe, when we are not tired or worried, our autonomic system rests at equilibrium, eliciting neither additional excitation (stimulating chemicals) nor relaxation (depressing chemicals). If this mode of balance were maintained, psychosomatic illnesses would not exist. But life poses a complicated array of continual dilemmas, and naturally we react. Because the way we feel reflects and is reflected by our body chemicals, we need not ingest any substance from outside our organisms to change our moods. Instead through the auto-pilot of the ANS, body hormones are called forth by the situations we find ourselves in (such as rush-hour traffic) and by various forms of recreation (TV programs), and most significantly by how we perceive and think. Modern habits of excess result in imbalance – we work too hard, we think too much, we overeat, we oversleep – the net effect of which taxes our ability to maintain equilibrium. When an overabundance of excitement occurs in one moment, the ANS eventually compensates by equalizing doses of depressant hormones, so that our organisms can (and often do) swing back and forth in response to what is commonly called "stress."

Drugs are agents that affect our nervous system in either one direction or the other. They can be natural hormones like adrenaline, which, if evoked excessively, cause problems such as mood swings and all types of psychosomatic disease, such as headaches, ulcers, heart attacks, and even cancer. Or they may be drugs that we administer from outside our bodies. Either kind can be detrimental. By introducing drugs from outside our body, we may further exacerbate the pendulum-like action in our body chemistry. Heroin depresses the Central Nervous System (CNS) as well as the ANS and our organism compensates down the road by natural body stimulation, which we experience as nervousness. Alcohol works this way too. The stimulant cocaine, used to offset sluggishness, eventually results in more sluggishness and progressively greater cravings for stimulation. This is the vicious cycle of addiction. It can occur by ingesting drugs or by eliciting our own body drugs through habits of excess (in action or even obsessional thinking patterns) that work either as stimulants or depressants. Marijuana, however, apparently doesn't affect the CNS.

> The Costa Rican study, edited by William E. Carter, specifically attempted to find such effects: "One of our principle objectives was to identify gross or subtle changes in major body and central nervous system functions which could be attributable to marijuana. We failed to do so. (Carter, 1980, p. 205)

As an example of the workings of this automatic mechanism: when a threat is perceived, fear is transmitted (via the Hypothalamus) to the body (through the ANS) as an order to prepare for strenuous action. Instantaneously, increased Sympathetic energizing pumps adrenaline-like chemicals throughout the organism. The heart rate increases dramatically, and the force of the heart beat becomes greater, to respond to additional needs of the body. More blood and oxygen is sent immediately to the brain and sense organs (eyes/ears/skin, etc.) for quicker perceptions and decisions. Stored sugars for energy are released by the liver. Capillaries of veins and arteries constrict, especially in the extremities, possibly so that the loss of blood from wounds will be minimized. Blood pressure rises because the veins and arteries have constricted. At the same time, the skeletal muscles constrict, almost in an armor-like protective fashion. Breath becomes fast, shallow, noisy and irregular in response to increased energy needs. The pupils of the eyes enlarge for clearer vision. The body has automatically become combat ready without our even knowing it. All we did was get frightened. The ANS did the rest. This body mode is appropriately called the "fight or flight" response (Benson, 1975, p. 23) and is a preparation solely for physical exertion. Once the action is over and the stimulant chemicals have been used, the organism rests at balance. But if no physical response takes place, which often happens in modern life, such as when we react to threats to our own status, ego, profit, etc. (as dangers), the body remains charged by the stimulating chemicals.

The ANS responds in the same way to reality or imagination. Just thinking fearful thoughts enjoins the combat mode through chemical outpourings, and then there is a strong instinctive need to rebalance body chemistry. Our organism is revved up but going nowhere, and we feel tense. The Parasympathetic side of the ANS reduces this tension by an equalizing excessive dose of depressant body chemicals, and then we may feel tired or sluggish. We cannot escape the law of balance. If we become overly excited at first, we become severely depressed later. Such chronic imbalance in the Autonomic System is defined as "stress," experienced physically as contraction or mentally as dissatisfaction, and it is responsible for most modern diseases.

Medicine for the Whole World

So many people, in all walks of life, from all social strata, in every country of the world, from the young to the old (for as long as there has been recorded history) have been and are now partakers of marijuana. They may have considered their enjoyment solely recreational without understanding that this magnificent natural remedy is actually and undeniably (in the strictest sense of the word) a medicine. It is "a substance used to treat disease," wherein disease is literally loss or lack of "ease" (which defines disruption of the entire person – body/mind/spirit). Marijuana as medicine is especially needed in today's stress-filled, fast-paced, competitive and insecure manner of daily living.

As the way marijuana works, in complete compatibility with the healthy functioning of all facets of humanness, becomes clear from the scientific presentation on the following pages, it is intended that the various, divided segments of the population espousing the employment of cannabis for different purposes will realize that medicinal, recreational, and sacramental utilization of this plant are actually identical. To be healthy is to be happy is to be holy, all of which are connected with cannabis use. Although modern life has divided up the three-fold nature of man and woman, in fact, there is no division. Our bodies are the temples of the Divine, to be kept in the utmost health, and our minds are the tools by which we recognize the essential values – if we are happy. The path of righteousness and happiness is the Medicine Path!

Although this book barely addresses the miraculous healing ability that hemp/marijuana can contribute to the deforestation, pollution and devastation of our dis-eased planet (see *The Emperor Wears No Clothes* and *Lifeline to the Future*), this fact must let us understand that the gift of nature in the form of a plant is a remedy, a holistic medicine of limitless extensions for healing the earth itself.

Those of us who know the truth have a choiceless commitment to expose it. Our commitment runs as deep as our souls. We enjoin you to further your knowledge and take your place among us.

Chapter 2 • The Physical Benefits
Marijuana and The Body's
Opposing Modes of Being

The wonder of marijuana is that it works in the body as an antidote to extreme swings. It does not stimulate. It does not depress. It does both at the same time, which is why it is unique, and so misunderstood by our scientific community educated from a narrow dualistic perspective.

> The most extensive study of marihuana, written nearly 100 years ago understood the complicated workings of marihuana, when it stated: "it is both sedative and stimulant." (Indian Hemp Drugs Commission, 1969, p. 491)

The simultaneous opposing action of marijuana is akin to balancing our entire system. Such balance in the ANS can be understood as a charged equilibrium, which is defined as "well-being," experienced as physiological expansion and psychological contentment and responsible for health. (See charts on pages 32 & 33.)

Many physiological changes occur with marijuana use, yet none of the changes is extreme in any one direction. The action of marijuana in the body causes slower and more expansive breathing (a direct result of Parasympathetic relaxation, which happens to us whenever we become relaxed). At the very same time, the alveoli (sacs in the lungs) expand, so that stale air is better eliminated, allowing for greater oxygen intake (a direct result of more Sympathetic participation, and which happens to us when we become excited), while both slower and deeper breathing occur, the depth of breath is even further aided by relaxing the "oppositional" muscles of the rib cage.

The rationale for health, underlying yogic postures, specifically addresses the benefits attained by increasing the size of the rib cage so as to accommodate an increased oxygen intake. Marijuana relaxes skeletal muscles (including the muscles that constrain the ribs). This efficient breathing has other far-reaching effects. Specifically, the brain receives more richly oxygenated blood and simultaneously receives a greater supply of that blood because of the dilation in all brain capillaries (increased Parasympathetic action). At the same time, because of an increase in Sympathetic energizing, the heart rate rises slightly to speed up further the distribution of more richly oxygenated blood. Heart rate increase is usually associated with an increased pulse rate because arteries and veins constrict with Sympathetic activity, but with marijuana no blood pressure rise occurs, since the capillaries have likewise expanded. In essence, the pump exerts a greater force and the enlarged pipes allow for greater flow. The net effect is a highly functioning, yet relaxed, system with better fuel. This is why, with marijuana, the feeling is both relaxed and alert, which explains, in part, the experience of being "stoned."

Normally the body vacillates between the two opposing modes of being. The effects of the complicated marijuana molecule somehow actually integrate these two modes, simultaneously, as absolutely nothing else does, except perhaps Anandamide–which also activates the Cannabinoid Receptors. When we examine the effects of marijuana within the framework of the body's healthy functioning, a dynamic interplay between either excitation or relaxation, we find that both the Relaxation Response and the Fight or Flight mode are elicited.

The extremes of these two modes are commonly referred to as bi-polarity in which one is either depressed or manic. Since marijuana creates no pendulum action, there is no possibility of it causing physical addiction. It is actually anti-addictive. This explains the mystery of so many regular marijuana users who claim that to stop using marijuana poses no problem, and it confirms all the scientific studies that report no addiction with marijuana. (The question of addiction to marijuana is further addressed in the Comentary: Questions and Answer section of the book.)

Marijuana has even been successful in treating alcoholics and morphine addicts, but the studies that demonstrated these results could not be replicated because of the government's ban on all marijuana testing by private agencies or medical scientists not employed by pharmaceutical companies.

Furthermore, the practice of smoking marijuana does not lead to addiction: From a limited observation on addicts undergoing morphine withdrawal...the impression was gained that marihuana had beneficial effects (George B. Wallace, MD, Chairman, From the Summary of Mayor LaGuardia's Committee,1944, p. 218).

Tod H. Mikuriya, MD, (1970) reports on successfully treating alcoholics with cannabis.

> ...the absence of any compelling urge to use the drug, the absence of any distressing abstinence symptoms, the statements that no increase in dosage is required to repeat the desired effect in users – justifies the conclusion that neither true addiction nor tolerance is found in marijuana users. (Mayor LaGuardia's Committee on Marijuana, 1944)

Although specific effects of marijuana in the body are well-known, each has been taken in isolation without noting that both sides of the Autonomic Nervous System are conjoined. Instead of a perspective that sees the whole person and the simple holistic effect of marijuana, a myopic and reductionistic method of measurement has been employed, and marijuana's profound meaning for health has been lost. Marijuana's action on the balancing mechanism of the human organism is extraordinary, perhaps because of the extreme complexity of the molecule and the uncanny perfect fit with specific receptor sites in the Hypothalamus (Howlett, 1990). It appears that by impacting on the ANS at its point of origin, above its locale of bifurcation in the body, marijuana resolves the "relaxation response" and the "fight or flight" reaction into one, thereby producing the subjective experience of unity. The literature concerning the experience of marijuana, from ancient to modern, is full of descriptions of "wholeness" or "oneness" – the paradox of the resolution of opposites.

OPPOSING MODES OF BEING
Vacillation Between Two Extremes

SYMPATHETIC OVERLOAD
"Fight or Flight"

PARASYMPATHETIC OVERLOAD
"Lethargic Depression"

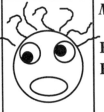

Manic

Beta Brainwaves

Muscles Tight

Pupils Dilated

Blood Pressure High

Heart Rate High

Mucus Membranes Dry

Bronchi Dilated

Veins/Arteries Constricted

Breathing: Fast, Shallow and Noisy

Muscles Relaxed

Pupils Constricted

Blood Pressure Low

Heart Rate Low

Mucus MembranesWet

Bronchi Constricted

Veins/Arteries Dilated

Breathing: Slow, Irregular, Noisy

Depressed

Theta Brainwaves

WITHOUT MARIJUANA
Patients can be overly excited or depressed
OUT OF BALANCE

THE MARIJUANA RESPONSE
Resolution of the Opposites

SYMPATHETIC • PARASYMPATHETIC BALANCE

Alpha Brainwaves

Alert and Relaxed

Muscles Relaxed

Pupils Constricted

Blood Pressure Slightly Lowered

Heart Rate Slightly Raised

Mucus Membranes Dry

Bronchi Dilated

Veins/Arteries Dilated

Breathing: Slow, Deep, Regular

WITH MARIJUANA
Patients are relaxed and energized
BALANCE IS RESTORED

Marijuana and the Brain

J ust as our Autonomic Nervous System is a two-fold process, so is our brain designed for dual action, with its left hemisphere and right hemisphere. Not surprisingly, these two sides are related to similar differences of action as in the autonomic system. The right side of the brain serves the receptive, creative, and nurturing experiences. We use this side during feelings connected to aesthetics, such as art and music, compassion, and global or spatial reasoning. In the area of cognition, this side adds to our understanding of meaning. The left hemisphere is geared toward linear, analytical, mechanical situations, such as mathematical problems; practical planning; and logical thought. Of course, both sides are always connected in constant communication with each other, and in dynamic complex cooperation. Yet different set and setting cause for greater emphasis in either one side or the other. This is called hemisphericity.

> It is...the idea that a given individual relies more on one mode or hemisphere than on the other. This differential utilization is presumed to be reflected in the individual's cognitive style – the person's preference – approach to problem solving. A tendency to use verbal or analytical approaches to problems, is seen as evidence of left-sided hemisphericity, while those who favor holistic or spatial ways of dealing with information are seen as right hemisphere people. (Springer and Deutsch, 1981, p. 239)

Where mechanical activities are constantly fostered, and where attention is geared to competition and acquisition, the workings of the left hemisphere predominate:

> Because we operate in such a sequential-seeming world and because the logical thought of the left hemisphere is so honored in our culture, we gradually damp out, devalue, and disregard the input of our right hemispheres. It's not that we stop using it altogether, it just becomes less and less available to us because of established patterns. (Prince, 1978, p. 58)

According to Deikman (1971), our most common mode of behavior is "attempting to manipulate the world around us ... through talking, pushing, grasping." He calls this the "hyper-aroused state of mind." The left side of the brain must overwork for most of us, most of the time, while the right brain is under-used, and therefore its special talents are neither appreciated nor cultivated. Studies describe right brain function as:

...silent, dark, intuitive, feeling, spatial, (and) holistic...does not require linear, structured analysis for its knowledge. (And we should note: the right hemisphere is also considered the feminine element, which emphasizes cooperation and nondomination). (Saraswati, 1984, p. 363)

In the materialistic world, such knowledge is basically devalued and denied, except perhaps in the arts. Appropriately, the right hemisphere also includes the creative flashes so often reported by geniuses: "The real thing is intuition. A thought comes and I may try to express it in words afterwards" (Einstein, 1954). But most people perceive an unreality and even irrationality about the intuitive faculty and feel a great skepticism of it.

Marijuana, by its effect on the ANS, enhances both sides of the brain. Through increased Sympathetic action, left brain perception is heightened while, at the same time, right brain reception is enhanced. This is a physiological fact. More blood, and cleaner blood, is sent to the brain as in the "fight or flight" reaction. And because of Parasympathetic dilation of all capillaries, which signifies relaxation, the blood supply of the entire brain is increased. More blood means more oxygen and consequently clearer and broader thinking. Since marijuana works on both sides of the brain, the most noticeable effect, in our fast-paced mind set, is one of slowing down, which blends the thrusting competitive attitude with the contrasting viewpoint of nurturance to arrive at a more cooperative balance. This experience is, however, not innate to marijuana, but to the mental set of the subject. When we are mellow, tired, and relaxed, marijuana is energizing and affords alertness, determination, and even strength. This variation in the physiological effects has caused great confusion from an either/or framework. And the balancing nature of marijuana (both/and) has not been understood. It both stimulates and relaxes, simultaneously, which equates to an unpredictable variation in effect that is solely dependent on the state of its subject. When the system is sluggish, as with natives in warm climates (Africa, India, South America), marijuana has been used extensively and for centuries to energize it.

A common practice among laborers...have a few puffs at a ganga [marihuana] pipe to produce well-being, relieve fatigue, stimulate appetite. (Chopra and Chopra, 1939, p.3)

When the system is hyper-aroused, as in today's lifestyle, marijuana calms. The significance of this fact cannot be ignored. It explains the increased creativity reported as a part of the marijuana experience, because when both sides of brain processes are heightened, both types of brain activity are greater. The left brain notices more, while the right brain receives more. This is the unification of logic and intuition. The term "expansion of consciousness" is explained physiologically as a "shifting of brain emphasis from one-sidedness to balance" (Sugerman and Tarter, 1978), which fits precisely with the feeling called "high."

Brain Synchronicity and Marijuana

Stress, as a chronic imbalance in the ANS, shows up as beta waves on an EEG machine and is experienced as worry. Marijuana ingestion has been shown to change the worried state by producing alpha waves, experienced as well being. This is a significant indication of balanced brain functioning because alpha waves occur when at least two waves from different brain loci are rising and falling in phase (in synchrony), as opposed to out-of-phase activity (when waves are nonsynchronous). "The EEG begins to report a higher percentage of alpha brain waves as soon as marijuana takes effect." (Ferguson, 1973, p. 114)

The brain waves calm down, and this signifies what scientists have termed "movement from an active to a receptive style" of being (Sugerman and Tarter, 1978, p. 84). This shift correlates with enhancement of all perceptual experiences, because mental clarity proceeds from a relaxed brain wave pattern by allowing thought processes to slow down. As the mind's busyness diminishes, the energy that is usually needed for rapid mental shifts is freed up and becomes available for more intense focusing in attention. Halikas et al. (1971) did a study with marijuana and concluded that enhancement of sense experience occurs "...as a direct consequence of slower rates of attentional shifts, and an increase of total energy – available to consciousness – manifested as intensification of (the contents of) consciousness."

Of course, an evening's marijuana use is not understood with any such analytical recognition. Instead, the felt sensation is of "moreness." In the fast lanes of modern life, where superficial and competitive relationships are all too common, the essence of humanness feels less. Marijuana, by its balancing effect, enriches this dimension of humanness.

Heart, Stomach and Lung Alteration

THE HEART: When we ingest marijuana, the heart swells through capillary enhancement, is fueled more by more fully oxygenated blood, while, at the same time, its contractions and expansions are greater, allowing for stronger pumping action to the rest of the body. In most cultures (ancient and modern), the heart center is designated as the "emotive vortex," which stands for the inner experience and outer expression of human love and affection. Generous and sympathetic people are said to have big hearts. During the marijuana experience this is literally the case and allows for the more full-bodied emotions that are in line with the claims of heightened feelings of love and compassion. Once the high is over, the heart is reduced to its usual size. But over a prolonged period, the heart muscle is known to become stronger for having been taxed for short periods. Jogging 20 minutes a day increases the strength of the heart, and to the extent that it is stronger, a jogger's heart displays a slower resting heart beat.

Although no studies have been done on the hearts of marijuana smokers, the odds are that they have stronger hearts too. It would be an easy study to accomplish, if the government would just allow tests to be conducted on a cross section of long term marijuana users and compare them to the already well-documented statistics of this same age/class disease profile, in this case, the incidence of heart disease. Psychiatric medicine has long realized that tension in the heart area indicates a defensive personality. The suppression of emotions, both tender and angry, is an attempt to ward off pain and puts the individual at risk of heart failure. Marijuana balances this chronic tension by its physiological action on the heart and its calming effects on the entire body.

THE STOMACH AND LUNGS: A tense stomach is the physical counterpart of mental tension and results in digestive problems (ulcers, colitis, stomach cancer, obesity, constipation, etc.). The mental tension is displayed through obsessing (or ruminating) over threats to one's welfare, resulting in excessive and continuous digestive messages (excessive Parasympathetic). As a cow chews its cud, or ruminates (always digesting in one of its four stomachs), so one who worries "eats" away at his or her innards. Psychologically, this implies an inability to let go of fear for oneself. Physiologically, the insecurity can be observed in the pattern and depth of the breath: "Shallow breathing can act as a personal defense against the experience of feeling" (Dychtwald, 1977, p.146).

Shallow breathing is noticed at the level of the stomach, because the diaphragm is the muscle of breath. If one does not breathe with the movement of the diaphragm, suppression of the breath takes place. Likewise, the stomach is stagnant. Over time, with continued "holding" or breathing contraction, the stomach loses its motility. This occurs as a response to feared situations, and to a greater or lesser degree becomes chronic in early years, in all populations where perfect balance is not encouraged:

> Very young children breathe with little inhibition or disturbance of natural breathing rhythms. But as one grows up, he (she) experiences traumas, imitates others, follows erroneous advice, and thereby develops incorrect breathing habits. These lead to chronic distortions in the breathing pattern and consequently to disequilibrium in other functions. Most adults breath irregularly or they chronically tense some of the muscles involved in the breathing process. (Ajaya, 1983, p. 196)

According to Rosenberg and Rand (1985):

> Breathing deeply and fully amplifies awareness of feelings. Many of the feelings that emerge with the deep breathing are uncomfortable, so most people avoid awareness by restricting their breathing. (p.107)

When the ANS becomes habituated to imbalance, as a direct result of chronic breathing distortion, the problem usually results from restricted exhalation. An organism that does not empty itself cannot refill. The term "anal retentive" describes the syndrome of being unable to "let go," or relax, as a habitual attitude toward life. Because of the complex interactions that occur throughout the body, once the breath is disturbed, various dysfunctions follow. In the digestive system, restriction of peristalsis results both from a subdued breath and skeletal muscular tension. Restriction in the exchange of carbon dioxide and oxygen, which attends with a shallow breath pattern, likewise adds to digestive disease as ANS functioning is skewed toward Sympathetic imbalance. The net result is nervousness (Sympathetic overload) or depression (Parasympathetic overload). Stomach problems correspond to ANS imbalance at either extreme. With Sympathetic overload, breathing imbalance results in diminished messages to the digestive system. Whereas with Parasympathetic overload, breathing imbalance results in excessive messages to the digestive system; either one of these overloads eventually results in an overload at the other extreme. Marijuana is an agent that can mitigate these extreme swings in the ANS. And therein is the reason that marijuana was, not so long ago, commonly prescribed for all sorts of digestive disturbances.

Patterns of shallow breathing have been studied to show that the less the body is supplied with superior oxygen, the less it is able to cope with threatening situations, physical or mental (Canon, 1932). Such shallow breathing is affected by chronically not breathing out sufficiently and is a direct result of restricted diaphragmatic movement. Inhalation, on the other hand, is secondary to exhalation, so that we breathe in, in direct correlation to the capacity exhaled. With asthma patients, who have trouble exhaling, marijuana facilitates exhalation:

> The fact that marijuana increases the diameter of bronchi in a manner unlike that of standard antiasthmatic agents makes its further investigation desirable. (Secretary of Health and Human Services, 1980, p.139; ibid., 1974, p.139)

Once the toxins in the lungs are more efficiently released, obtaining sufficient oxygen by deep and full breathing follows automatically. As rigidity in the body is released or reduced by the action of marijuana, there is a corresponding reduction of mental tension that translates into a feeling of expansion and well-being and explains the reverential attitude commonly expressed by marijuana lovers.

LEGAL MARIJUANA RECIPIENTS
Under the Federal *Compassionate Care Protocol* Program

Because it balances bodily processes, marijuana alleviates many disease symptoms that conventional aggressive one-sided drugs cannot. Under the *Compassionate Care Protocol* program, government-grown marijuana is distributed to the eight seriously ill patients in the United States. There are many other gravely ill persons who actually passed the walls of red-tape required to be admitted to the program, however these patients were denied access in 1991 when President Bush closed the program because Marijuana Therapy was becoming too well-known.

Each of the persons listed suffers from a disability that marijuana makes less difficult to endure. Some can walk because of it, some don't hemorrhage anymore, some can stand the pain, and some can see, but not one of them can understand what their government is trying to accomplish by denying this medicine. Those patients I was able to contact were enthusiastic about having their names and phone numbers listed so that they can be contacted for information and questions.

1. Barbara Douglass, Iowa   (712) 732-2929
2. George McMahon, Iowa   (515) 379-2808
3. Corrine Millet, Nebraska   (402) 721-6077
4. Elvy Musikka, Florida   (954) 981-1225
5. Robert Randall, D.C.   Not Available
6. Irvin Rosenfeld, Florida   (800) 255-2943
7. Chris Woiderski, Florida   Not Available
8. Unknown Patient

Chapter 3 • Psychological Benefits
Perceiving: Sense Organs

As the body's workings can become more harmonious with marijuana, the functioning of the five senses can be noticeably improved. This naturally occurs as the organs of sense are fueled with more oxygenated blood, as well as being less constrained or constricted. The eyes, the ears, the skin, the nose, and the taste buds are supplied with more and better "fuel" during the marijuana experience. There is nothing mysterious or mystical about the subjective feelings that all marijuana users report, such as: finer appreciation of visual and auditory stimuli (art and music); more enhanced sense of taste and appetite; greater feelings of tenderness and eroticism (sex is better); and a deeper and more insightful understanding of all experience, including our own thoughts and emotions.

> Appetite is regulated by the hypothalamus, where marihuana works directly. This is parasympathetic energizing, which aids sugar storage [i.e., takes it out of our blood stream and saves it in the liver], and is therefore responsible for appetite increase. Owing to a greater supply of oxygenated blood to the taste buds [Parasympathetic], there is greater appreciation and enjoyment of food. Stimulants [such as cocaine] release our body's supply of stored sugars [which depletes us] into the blood stream and kills our appetite. Of course, the taste buds constrict with all body excitement, and therefore food is less enjoyable.
> Grass [marihuana]…heightens your enjoyment of your perceptions and conceptions…[It] causes the feeling of just being alive…There are four areas in which this heightening of the sexual response is clearly manifest; foreplay, control, orgasm, creativity. (Margolis and Clorfene, 1970, p. 57)

This enhanced capacity of all the body's sense organs (including the sense one has of him/herself) accounts for the mental interpretation of intense perceptions, known as the "high." Technically speaking, this is really a (marvelous) side effect to balancing the ANS. In our discussion, the trigger to the high experience is marijuana, but many other activities can also produce it, such as jogging, chanting, fasting, isolation, meditation, and prayer. Life's precious moments represent entry to the "high," such as the birth of a child, the rediscovery of romance, and even witnessing a beautiful sunset.

Altered states of consciousness can be triggered by hypnosis, psychedelics, deep prayer, sensory deprivation, acute psychosis, sleep deprivation, fasting, epileptic attacks and migraines, hypnotic monotony, electronic brain stimulation, alpha training, clairvoyance, muscle relaxation, isolation, photic stimulation, kundalini yoga. (Ferguson, 1973, p. 55)

Another component to the intensification of sensory perceptions and mental understanding can be understood by the equilibrium marijuana produces in brain functioning. The marijuana experience is innately connected to the mental set and environmental setting of the subject. As we have seen, marijuana works toward equalizing ANS energizing, which in our fast-paced world will be toward receptivity and away from the striving, grasping, hurried, and active mode of being. When this takes place, our rate of attentional shifting also slows down. The energy that it takes to maintain the active, aggressive mode is therefore likewise freed up:

One of the most commonly reported effects of marijuana is the enhancement of perceptual experiences: auditory, gustatory, tactual, olfactory...visual experiences are reported as occurring in a more intense fashion.

These phenomena are expected as a direct consequence of slower rate of attentional shifts, and they may be supported by an increase in total energy... if not used to produce attentional shifts is available to consciousness.(Halikas, Goodwin, and Guze 1971)

The great sense of insight produced by marijuana is also explained by Sugerman and Tarter (1978) as resulting from a slower rate of shifting one's attention, thereby in the act of "thinking," the thoughts "will be imbued with enhanced intensity."

Another faculty, sometimes called the sixth sense, is our undeveloped capacity for perceiving the world and its meaning. This is the dimension of intuition, or deeper-than-usual understanding with which poets and saints are familiar. The marijuana user becomes aware of this sense. Many artistic and creative people claim this as the single most beneficial aspect of using marijuana.

Although most scientific authors who present new respectable evidence for the harmlessness of marihuana use make no claim for its surprising usefulness. I do make that claim: Marihuana is a catalyst for specific optical and aural aesthetic perceptions. I appreciate the structure of certain pieces of jazz and classical music in a new manner under the influence of marihuana, and these apprehensions have remained valid in years of normal consciousness. (Ginsberg, 1966, p. 107)

Development of the sixth sense merges with, harkens, and even hastens, spiritual development, and may easily lead to reverence for the plant that brings this radiance:

The Report of the Indian Hemp Drugs Commission, conducted by the Indian and Great British Governments, was the most extensive examination of marihuana to date. Some of the significant statements from that massive work, which represented the entire Indian cultural orientation over the course of its 5000-year-intact civilization concerning the reverent attitude toward marihuana include:

> To the Hindu, the hemp plant is holy...a guardian lives in the marihuana leaf...its thought bracing qualities show...[It] is the home of the great Yogi ...its powers give [ganja] a high place among lucky objects...Oaths are taken on its leaf...spirit of bhang (marihuana) is the spirit of freedom and knowledge...[is] the cleanser of ignorance ...students of the scriptures at Benares are given bhang [marihuana and milk beverage] before they sit to study, [to] center their thoughts on the Eternal. (Indian Hemp Drugs Commission, 1969, p. 492)

Mental Balance

The novice cannot fully appreciate the marijuana experience, since it takes time to realize the association between heightened capacities and cannabis. Yet the mental states that occur with pot are neither unfamiliar nor mysterious. Although the naturally occurring brain hormone Anandamide has just been discovered, its effects have always been part of the human experience. These effects are subtle and for that reason scientists have not even known to search for it. Only because of the THC encoding of the cannabinoid receptor in the brain did it become clear that the brain, itself, must have its own key. That is why none of the changes of the marijuana experience taken separately are different from what we experience every day.

> It is striking that so many...medical reports failed to mention any intoxicating properties of (marijuana). Rarely, if ever, is there any indication that patients – hundreds of thousands must have received cannabis in Europe in the nineteenth century – were "stoned" or changed their attitudes toward work, love, their fellow man, or their homelands. (Tart, 1975, p. 153)

Instead, it is the totality of the subtle changes that are notable and noticed, but noticed only after one focuses attention:

Typically the first few times a person smokes marijuana...the overall pattern of his consciousness stays quite ordinary and he (or she) usually wonders why others make so much fuss. (ibid., p.154)

Natural feelings of expansion that correspond to favorable perceptions, such as a sense of accomplishment, are experiences common to us all. What makes marijuana unique and beneficial is its ability to summon these states of well-being at will. Anandamide may well be blocked from being secreted effectively or received appropriately once the organism has become habituated to disequilibrium. By resummoning the lost ability to gain balance through the marijuana experience, the bliss of life may be reawakened. From such a positive point of view, problems are understood and more easily resolved when tranquility is coupled with insight. The regular marijuana user reaches these states of tranquility over and over again, leading to a fuller integration of the person with his/her environment.

According to Abraham Maslow(1968), who developed a theoretical framework to measure high-functioning adults, or as he termed them "self-actualizers," certain, few members of a society reach a more mature or "more fully human" state as a way of life. His paradigm presents a hierarchy of goals for the developing individual, with "basic human needs" as only the first stage to be mastered along an ascension that culminates in "meta motives" or goals of a higher, more artistic, less self-centered, more individualistic nature. Self-actualizers are those who have gratified basic needs and are, therefore, no longer motivated by them. Instead higher motivations are their goals. Self actualizers represent a small percentage of society who exhibit greater degrees of health and joy than is common for most people. However, according to Maslow, virtually everyone has had an exalted, expanded period of consciousness triggered by "music/beauty/luck." These times of happiness and well-being he terms "peak experiences" and notes that they are usually forgotten, since no importance is attached to them. We might suggest that those hundreds of millions of people around the world who use marijuana to experience higher levels of life, do so specifically because of the great import they ascribe to being "high", i.e., feeling better, happier, more expansive, and therefore, more tolerant and compassionate.

Although we commonly refer to the body, mind, and spirit as separate entities, these divisions do not really exist. The roots, branches, and leaves serve the same purpose when we are discussing different facets of tree-ness. But to appreciate the concept of tree, the entire entity must be considered. No one would ever logically argue that the leaves exist separate from branches or roots, or that the health of the leaves is not innately connected to the health of the roots. Holistic health is a return to a basic age-old notion of wholeness that existed throughout history. It views a person in the same fashion that a botanist sees a tree. It is "all of a piece," and any division that is allowed is done so for the sole purpose of simplifying discussion. We can see, then, that as the body's modus operandi is altered during the marijuana experience, the mind's processes likewise change.

The Psychological Marijuana Experience

Accepting that psychological defense mechanisms correspond to body tension, obviously it doesn't matter in what sphere the alteration begins, since they are two sides of the same coin and therefore affect each other completely. According to Elmer Green:

> Every change in the physiological state is accompanied by an appropriate change in the mental-emotional state, conscious or unconscious...and conversely, every change in the mental-emotional state, conscious or unconscious is accompanied by an appropriate change in the physiological state. (Ferguson, 1973, p. 27)

When the body relaxes, so does the mind. But releasing tension and inhibitions via drunkenness or tranquilization is accompanied by numbing this normal consciousness, leading to a state of unawareness. Whereas marijuana results in an "altered state of consciousness," the depressant drugs have been described as producing "altered states of unconsciousness" (Sugerman and Tarter, 1978, p. 291) allowing for relaxation without awareness.

As a consequence of the capacity of individual thought, each of us maintains a personal unconsciousness, which comprises repressed issues that often contradict the image we have of ourselves. The unconscious mind can be exposed in dreams or by drinking alcohol to excess. It can reveal itself in psychoanalysis, meditation, and during the marijuana experience, as well as in times of extreme stress (as in nervous breakdown), and during life-threatening experiences. The unconscious is exposed by breaking down the barrier between it and the conscious mind. This barrier is commonly called "defense mechanisms" or "armour" by Western psychology, so named by the the famed psychologist Wilhelm Reich. The healthiest person is depicted as one who has very few defense mechanisms that shield him/her from unsavory aspects of the hidden personality. It follows that the healthy person will not need to invest much energy in keeping out unconscious motives/fears/memories from conscious awareness and will be therefore more broad-minded, or as they say, "less defended." In the field of psychology, optimum health implies total vulnerability to all facets of personality, where the unconscious blends with the conscious to form an "integrated" person. Carl Jung (1986) explained it as a blending of the "persona" (outward personality) with the "shadow" (or internal side of human nature), so that nothing of the self remained in the dark – hidden from awareness.

Marijuana exposes things. When used over a period of time, it allows us to witness our many subtle motives which, under normal consciousness, are usually not noticeable. The experience of marijuana seems to open the curtain to our self-deceptions, and gives us access to our innermost private agendas. "Alcohol primarily relieves anxiety and promotes optimism. It makes the society and what one has to do with society OK. Pot, on the other hand, turns you inside yourself" (Freidenberg).

The traditional Western modality of treating neurosis has a director or outer authority as the witness (in the form of the therapist). Neurosis is understood as the dark, dangerous side of ourselves that conflicts with our attitudes and ideals, but with which everyone must somehow come to terms, if he/she is to become whole. Rejection of the dark side is the neurotic "division in personality, and hostility between conscious or unconscious." (Rosenberg, et al., 1985, p. 309) In the more liberal Transpersonal Psychology (adapted from Eastern Theory), the "patient" becomes a student and attends to his/her own conflicts, as in meditation or yoga. Self-responsibility is the main difference between the two schools of psychology. In yoga psychology one needs to learn on one's own, rather than be shown by an authority representing the fuel for change. Meditation is the ultimate tool for self-knowledge. In the East, marijuana has been used to facilitate the process for millennia:

> Cannabis plays a very significant role in the meditative ritual used to facilitate deep meditation and heighten awareness...use of hemp is likewise so common now [1979] in this region [Tibet] that the plant is taken for granted as an everyday necessity. (Schultes and Hofmann, 1979, p. 99)

It was just this catalytic effect of marijuana – to expose the unconscious and increase the patient's vulnerability, while maintaining awareness and understanding – that prompted psychologists (in the 60s and 70s) to utilize marijuana extensively in the therapeutic studies before the government ban. Understanding one's motives over time, and with active registration, serves to encourage the ability to look past usual defensive positions.

Optimum psychological health ("ego strength") is evidenced by full integration of the unconscious within the realm of awareness: "the problem is simply to open the channels between the conscious and unconscious minds" (Weil). It can also be realized as accepting or loving (all of) oneself totally without judgement.

Anything that enhances the functioning of the body mitigates mental tension as well, and with a "witnessing" aspect, there exists the possibility of learning and growth within the personality. Loosening of defense mechanisms automatically changes the notion of the self or (I-ness), since awareness expands to include repressed fears and forgotten needs. At times, the experience of seeing ourselves in an unfavorable light can be painful. At other times, when we are not focused on our shortcomings, a less defended viewpoint frees up the energy that maintained the repression. The experience of the NOW is intensified, because of the increased psychic energy available to perceive the moment. This intensification is the summation of all the effects that have accrued to the entire body-mind. When it (the high) occurs with marijuana, much of its emphasis is due to the immediacy of the change. Enhanced sense perception (including the mental sense of oneself) occurs as soon as the marijuana takes effect – within just a few minutes, if smoked, and within an hour, if ingested. It is like suddenly operating without resistance (such as, muscle-armor, or mental-tension) and implies a gentler outlook than is usual. This explains why marijuana is associated with peace rather than aggression and probably explains the worry of detractors who claim a loss of "the competitive spirit" with cannabis use:

> Marijuana is symbolic of a more passive, contemplative and less competitive attitude toward life than has been traditional in the U.S. It is usually denounced by people who like things the way they are. (Snyder, 1972, p. 128)

The balanced personality (of "extreme health") has not been studied by traditional psychology, which up to now has focused on the conflicts of neurotic populations. In the 1960s and 70s, with the emergence of the Humanistic psychologies, formal theory developed to include health as a natural progression in human growth (See Maslow, May, Tart, Ornstein). Holistic health (with its emphasis on wellness rather than sickness) is an outgrowth of this orientation. Its goal is balance, as contrasted with suppressing the symptoms of illness (imbalance). The methods are varied, but always include self-regulation and responsibility on the part of the student, reduction of tension through healthy relaxation methods, and replacement of dysfunctional breathing patterns.

> We have been able to confirm repeatedly Wilhelm Reich's observation that psychological resistance and defenses use the mechanism of restricting the breathing. Respiration has a special function among the physiological functions of the body. It is an autonomous function, but it can easily be influenced by volition, increase of the rate and the depth of breathing typically loosens the psychological defenses and leads to release and emergence of the unconscious (and superconscious) material. (Grof, 1988, p.171)

Less tense populations tend toward greater appreciation of the moment, are less apt to accept a hurried way of life, and more prone to creative pursuits. This accounts for the widespread use of marijuana among artists, musicians, and populations less interested in power and more interested in self-expression and human relationship. It also probably explains why very competitive and rigid people are so against the marijuana experience, since these personality types are innately anxious and suspicious of change. Imbalance becomes fixed, familiar, and even comfortable, whereas balance is feared as the unknown.

With marijuana, balance is especially startling, because it occurs quickly and effortlessly. This effect alone is most likely responsible îor the fear of the "work ethic" against marijuana. To arrive at a feeling of well-being without hard work or pain seems immoral in the West. This arises from the foolish notion that happiness (or wellness) is unnatural, even sinful, and is based on accentuated alienation from the "whole" of life. On the other hand, a holistic orientation envisions higher states of happiness as the natural birthright of human beings.

Marijuana Benefits are Long Term

The benefits of marijuana are far ranging, long term, and not as instantaneous as the "high." In the short run the equilibrium that occurs is only temporary and reverses as soon as the "high" wears off. Conscious realization of one's hidden motives and defenses is not effortless, but includes emotional pain. The marijuana experience itself does not miraculously cure. Instead it allows the body a respite from the tensions of imbalance, while exposing the mental confusion of the mind. Although, in the short run, balance is easily lost, the essential tendency to homeostatic habituation (health) develops over time. In the long run, then, marijuana can serve as the vehicle by which the body-mind heals itself. This is not to suggest that all one needs to do is smoke pot to dissolve the illness of years. What takes place, instead, is subtle and long term. With the expansiveness that occurs with marijuana, the subject may begin to notice infinite possibilities to raise the quality of his/her life that would otherwise have remained hidden from normal, defensive consciousness. And feelings of health and happiness naturally lead to hope, which of itself can be curative.

The marijuana experience of balance becomes a learned and, over time, somewhat permanent, response as the essential human tendency to homeostasis is reawakened and the natural healing process restored. A person who breathes, thinks, and feels healthier for a short time, with no adverse consequence, (discounting the discomfort that may accompany fuller awareness) is certainly better off for the experience. And if persons habitually breathe, think, and feel healthier, through meditation, marijuana, vegetarianism or what have you, they begin to face toward health, whether or not they continue any particular practice. In other words, it is better to have used marijuana and stopped, than never to have used it at all. But of course, it is best to use marijuana regularly:

> Any process or method that helps defuse the toxicity of a stressful event or situation is good. (Wallace, 1989)

Mental Imbalance

A deep sense of insecurity exists in most lives. The sadness of death perhaps never completely loses its influence over us. We develop all kinds of conscious and unconscious anxieties associated with that aversion. Oftentimes, these influence us, buried as they are like a basement furnace that keeps everything warm without a visible flame. Awareness of such fears is discouraged, for it causes pain. Defenses keep these insecurities hidden beneath a facade of competence and/or confidence, creating the neurotic personality. The amount of fear, and how successfully it is repressed, determines the vulnerability of a particular subject to a state of "paranoia." The more we have a deluded sense of self-esteem, the greater the possibility for panic. Another way of understanding paranoid reactions is from an energetic model. As the conscious mind habitually represses unconscious motives, energy to do so can be likened to a dam that holds back the floodwater. The slightest break in the dam signals a lessening of the holding strength, which consequently loosens the floodgates. Marijuana can act as the loosening agent, so that whatever has been banned from consciousness may come cascading forth. To uncover our deceptions without our usual rationalizations can be unpleasant, an experience that has turned many psychologically fragile individuals away from marijuana despite its therapeutic catharsis.

Predictably, if we continue to unleash that which is repressed, deep-seated fears can be worked out and resolved. Just as when a dam is dismantled, the floodwater no longer holds power but is instead merged in the larger river, so too does insecurity lose its strength to manipulate us unawares, when it is incorporated into conscious recognition. With awareness, conflict can be dealt with, allowing us greater freedom in action.

Almost everyone has learned what life's expectations are by the time they are three or four years old. Already by that age a certain "cluster of tendencies" – certain desires or feelings have been subdued in order to attain/maintain approval and love. The more we need love (or feel unloved), the more we strive toward the ideal image that we have internalized in our earliest years. Accepting and adopting standards of behavior is the process of "civilizing" that all healthy and energetic children resist, in one way or another. As development progresses, this "cluster of hidden tendencies" takes on an entity of its own. It becomes the shadow of the front presented to the world. The front is Jung's "persona" whom the outside world can see. What is invisible is the shadow: all that has been chronically denied as we ascend the ladder to neurotic maturity and adulthood.

Regardless of the model used, marijuana resolves conflict by de-emphasizing extreme aggressiveness and stroking the receptive sides of human nature. This unification or balance, however, may be responsible for changes in goals and values. It is the healthy balancing nature of marijuana that is most beneficial to the individual and most threatening to modern society. According to Bromberg:

> [The Protestant ethic]...in this country condemns marijuana as an opiate used solely for pleasure (whereas) alcohol is accepted because it lubricates the wheels of commerce and catalyzes social intercourse...marijuana's effect in producing a state of introspection and bodily passivity is repellant to a cultural tradition that prizes activity, aggressiveness, and achievement. (Mayor LaGuardia's Committee, 1944, p. 203)

Social Imbalance

Our entire society may be viewed as one of denial, fearful of unspoken and unresolved issues. The fear of drug use, without an understanding of its basic cause, its function, and its deeply felt need explains today's mindset. If we examine the Systems Theory in psychology, this can be more clearly understood. Any system, be it a family, an office group, or a society may operate dysfunctionally. As a repressed family is sick and naturally influences its children in the direction of its imbalance, so does a civilization that is operating from disequilibrium produce a citizenry that is sick. "The addiction [imbalance] is catching" (Schaef, 1987).

We need just to look at the unwholesome food/programs/drugs

that are our daily bread, to realize the universality of the cultural imbalance. We learn to breathe, think, and eat within the structure of our life situation. Our modern culture has been similarly called materialistic, denying, or competitive. Our citizens die of cancer, heart attacks, and hypertension – all of which can be classified as diseases of disequilibrium, directly compatible with Sympathetic Overload, which manifests as competition, and is called stress. The overlay of today's values are skewed in the direction of acquisition, born of an attitude of fear and protectiveness. Our children are immediately taught that being smart is eminently more important than being fair. To be "number one," i.e., to gain financial success by overpowering other people's productivity, vision, and determination, is the American Dream. Intrinsic human values are given lip-service, but nowhere in our educational system are our children taught to look inward so as to develop a core of principles and a systematic method to realize them. Instead, we bombard our children's intellects with ever-faster computer games, programs for the gifted, continuous TV, and constant activities, all of which aid acceleration of linear thought. To accommodate to this mode of living, everyone is necessarily "geared up," or stimulated. Anything that slows down the process is devalued or denied. So while marijuana can help to rebalance the personality, through direct, measurable benefits to the psychological/physical organism, such an effect threatens the social agenda.

The citizens who cannot cope become the sacrifice. They are often the hardest working, fastest living, stoic types who develop cancer or die suddenly from heart failure. Their mechanical orientation cannot be changed by whim or will. They are who they are, and they represent the very striving by which the society fuels itself. To maintain the culture's status quo, health and happiness must be compromised. Ironically, marijuana, so beneficial to the balance of the body and peace of the mind, seems to endanger the very core of capitalism. "Drugs of unconsciousness" (especially alcohol) which anesthetize the psychological pain, and block out the causes of a repressive society, are much more acceptable. The fact that in the long run they destroy many lives needs to be overlooked because they don't interfere with the overall values of society and are relied upon by many "respectable" addicts to relieve their internal stress, especially severe in industrialized societies.

The social paranoia that marijuana has met with is surely under-standable. To a society skewed toward constant pressure, the idea of slowing down is frightening. The observation has often been made that the use of marijuana "kills ambition," "makes us sleepy," and generally makes us less concerned with worldly goings-on. "It slows me down" is the often heard complaint, or just as often, "I get sleepy." A comparison to the Western viewpoint on pain is appro-priate. Take a pill —never mind searching out the source of the problem. Subdue the symptom – ignore the cause – and even deny the foolhardiness of such a philosophy. Marijuana is an agent that balances the Autonomic Nervous System. Is it possible that the "slowing down" and the nap are the organism's turning toward health? A relaxed attitude is only harmful to the goals of a workaholic. Excessive competition feeds stress and cannot be the healthiest and happiest way to live. Then the argument turns to, "If everyone smoked pot, would the whole world stop functioning?" The world would certainly not fall apart, even if, by some miracle, everyone did smoke pot. Imagine the possibilities for cooperation throughout the world that might take place, if everyone somehow had a slightly higher consciousness that included "you as well as me." Of course, from an acquisitive position, this would be quite unprofitable. Nevertheless, the higher values of nonaggression are always present somewhere in the human psyche, as difficult as they may be to retrieve. Study upon study has shown that less violence is associated with marijuana use than any legal drug used for recreation.

> Marijuana is much less likely than alcohol to produce aggressive behavior. Neither the marijuana user nor the drug itself can be said to constitute a danger to public safety. For, whatever an individual is, in all of his (and her) cultural, social and psychological complexity, is not going to vanish in a puff of marijuana smoke. (Mayor LaGuardia's Committee, 1944)

Just as significantly, in exact opposition to much maligning of marijuana, all studies support the fact that nothing important is ever forgotten or neglected because of the use of marijuana. People can drive, take care of their children, write legal briefs, perform mean-ingfully at their jobs, and just as brilliantly at their studies, if they are regular marijuana users. Marijuana does not debilitate one's behavior, as alcohol/tranquilizers/speed/cocaine do. From the Secretary of Health and Human Services (1980):

> In the politicized and emotionally charged atmosphere surrounding marihuana use, far too much research has been marred by the predetermined stance of the researchers. Much that claims to be research is barely above polemics. Fully aware of this problem, we tried to look as objectively as possible at the consequences of long term heavy use. We employed natural, as well as clinical settings, used an unprecedented number of carefully matched subjects. Our measures were as thoughtfully chosen as we could make them. None of us who directed the project had any preconceived notions as to what we might find. We were entering a new field of research and were willing and anxious to accept any data or insights that might emerge.
>
> Many of us were frankly surprised that we were unable to uncover any real consequences of prolonged use....Indeed, some ...were sincerely disappointed at the lack of significant differences between our controlled population of uses and nonusers.
>
> But no findings in science are in themselves findings, indeed findings of the most important type. For years, those of us who made up the research team had assimilated the pseudo-scientific reports of the popular press to the effects that marihuana use, over time, could lead to a frightening array of deleterious effects. We had frankly expected to find at least some of these in our research. Yet the fact, that we did not is entirely in keeping with results of the only other serious studies of chronic effects in which intervening socio-cultural variables have been properly controlled, namely, those studies carried out in Greece and Jamaica. Had we looked at almost any other substance, alcohol, for instance, we would have found more effects than we found with marihuana.... Overall the findings indicated that the level of marihuana has little influence on performance in neuropsychological intelligence, and personality battery. (Carter, 1980, p. 187)

Mayor LaGuardia's Committee also confirmed this lack of deleterioius effects:

> The publicity concerning the catastrophic effects of marihuana smoking in New York City is unfounded...the marihuana users accustomed to daily smoking for a period of from two and a half to sixteen years, showed no abnormal system functioning which would differentiate them from non-users. There is definite evidence in this study that the marihuana users were not inferior in intelligence to the general population and that they had suffered no mental or physical deterioration as a result of their use of the drug...The use of marihuana does not lead to morphine or heroin or cocaine addiction and no effort is made to create a market for these narcotics by stimulating the practice of marihuana smoking. (1944)

According to Sugerman & Tarter:

> Should memory be sampled under the influence of marihuana, it could be done with greater intensity and with a greater flow of deeper-lying or unusual associations being brought into consciousness...Nevertheless, virtually all studies completed to date (late 1979) show no evidence of chronically impaired neuropsychologic test performance in humans at dose level experimentally studied...In a study of chronic Greek users, a different technique was employed to determine whether brain atrophy might be present in heavy users. The findings were negative: that is, users were not found to differ from non-users in evidence of gross brain pathology. (1988, p. 286)

The truth is the majority of people do not use marijuana to revolutionize their way of life. Instead, they enjoy its physiological relaxant effect unawares, and appreciate the sense of mental well-being that accompanies the experience. Depending upon the variety of marijuana (sativa or indica), this sense of well-being has subtle variations; especially in Homeopathic medical treatment, in the 19th century and early 20th century, differences between the two strains were recognized.

When it first became popular in the West, marijuana was imported mainly from tropical zones, where the sativa strain of cannabis is indigenous. This type of marijuana is known for its "cerebral high," having little noticeable body participation. No studies concerning the different effects of sativa vs. indica have been done, but from the lack of physical sensation, it is reasonable to assume more Sympathetic or stimulant qualities in sativa than indica (a cooler climate type). This is compatible with the notion that in hotter climates, less calming is desirable from a recreational substance, since hot climates in themselves cause lethargy. Many connoisseurs of marijuana prefer the sativa high, although in the last decade it has become very scarce due to domestic cultivation of strains that thrive in temperate zones. "Cerebral highs" are experienced as lightness of thought beyond usual concern with self-esteem. In relationships, a cerebral high attunes the participants to a less separate sense of others. Conversation is animated and a general feeling of comraderie is in the air.

The indica strain of cannabis offers more of the "body high." Depth rather than height best describes the subjective experience. Rather than freedom in the mind, the felt sensation is freedom of the body. This state more closely mimics deep relaxation. Thought patterns do not approach the clarity of thought of a "cerebral high." In contrast, the "body high" is similar to the reverie that precedes sleep. While thinking may be diminished, more sensitivity to non-verbal experiences, such as music and color, comes into play. Physiologically, a true "body high" probably is the result of more Parasympathetic input. Participants often become quieter, since internal silence predominates.

Indica thrives in temperate areas, and as such it has become more popular with the American marijuana farmer. It is a shorter variety, thus it is more suited for the limits of indoor gardens and comes to fruition earlier in outdoor gardens. In less tropical zones, recreational substances are compatible with tempering the bustle usual to cooler climate cultures. As horticultural interest has grown, a cross between the indica and sativa "species" of cannabis has given the modern marijuana user the subtleties of both strains. Nowadays quality marijuana, grown in the U.S., is usually a hybrid of indica and sativa varieties.

Marijuana and Mental Processes

Marijuana will not tolerate repression. Tranquilizers and depressants relax the body and release tension, but the state of mind associated with these drugs is "unconsciousness" whereby we escape rather than resolve our dilemmas. Alcoholism is an extreme need of both the body and personality periodically to release the nervousness that has accumulated and continues to accumulate to an unbearable degree. It serves the same function for the collective personality of the society, as well. A culture in which alcohol and tranquilizers are the prevalent form of release prefers not to witness internal confusion and actually chooses to act without conscious participation, maintaining a semi-numb condition. One feels less pressure, expresses less emotion and is less able to care – all as a consequence of being less conscious. This type of relaxation releases conflict without knowledge of its source, treating the symptom while ignoring the cause. The uncovering of inner confusion, so prominent with marijuana, is conspicuously absent with depressants. As the overall benefits of insightfulness obtained from its use lead to a greater freedom, marijuana is shunned by individuals who need a status quo in the personality or social position.

Sigmond Freud developed and expounded the understanding that we mechanically base our actions on programs devised throughout life, and many esoteric schools, ancient and modern, have taught the same. Being aware of these programs is very difficult, since ordinary consciousness has within it the conspiracy to keep the mind comfortable and free of conflict. This operates collectively, as well as individually. Whenever confronted, this usual state of mind automatically assumes a defensive posture by relying on distorted rationalizations, which are evident in a repressive and intolerant social order. By contrast, the open and aware consciousness often leads to spiritual realizations, irrelevant in mainstream thinking. In today's world this understanding is uncommon. Higher morals and ethics, as propounded by organized religions, are agreed upon by the masses, especially during church attendance, but are otherwise too difficult to maintain when personal survival is at stake. Universal spiritual values, so often released with marijuana, can break down the conditioned defensive mentality.

It appears as if society, as well as the programmed, individual mind, needs to hold in check the notion that we love our neighbor as ourselves. There is no way that we can love our neighbor as ourselves, nor any way that our economy can subscribe to a policy of cooperation, when the very life of business enterprise is dependent upon "profit first and foremost." Cooperation within free enterprise is a difficult reality so long as "me first" remains the primary motivation. A neurotic society, with its deeply imbedded habit of maladaptive coping methods, is resistant to change. Marijuana can be of tremendous benefit in exposing the distorted perspectives responsible for social, class, and racial conflict. It can open the "doors of perception," and thereby alter the very core of the personality, by allowing a view of the transcendent values of human life.

> Cannabis is anathema to the dominant culture because it deconditions or decouples users from accepted values. When pursued as a lifestyle [it] places a person in intuitive contact with less goal oriented and less competitive behavior patterns. For these reasons marijuana is unwelcome in the modern office environment, while a drug such as coffee, which reinforces the

values of industrial culture, is both welcomed and encouraged.
(McKenna, 1992, p. 155)

It diminishes the power of the ego, has a mitigating effect on
competition, causes one to question authority, and reinforces the
notion of the merely relative importance of social values. (ibid.,
p.165)

Psychosomatic Disease

Stress related disorders are commonly referred to as being psychosomatic, which is a simplified way of saying that, in the case of
cancer for instance, it affects and is affected by both the body and
mind. In other words, except for some children's cancer, and except
for environmental mishaps (as in Chernobyl or over exposure to
specific carcinogens), cancer is a disease of, and an outgrowth from,
the whole person. In such a framework, the question of responsibility for one's illness is often raised, almost as though the patient is to
blame or deserves to be sick. This judgement is faulty in that it fails
to appreciate the wholeness out from which a person's psychological and physiological tendencies have been forged.

Beginning with excessive conscious and unconscious interpreta-
tions of danger (as a result of dysfunctional upbringing, immersion
in unhealthy lifestyles – including too fast a pace of life, the wrong
diet, and obsession with material success – the life-sustaining
systems of the entire organism become habitually turned away from
relaxation, calmness, and expansion. Combat-ready habituation is
a "whole" person agenda, most noticeably measurable as an abundance of stimulants (ANS imbalance) but also including suppression of ordinary immunological responses.Such a state defines the
entire person in the same way that the totality of environmental
influences are measured by scores on I.Q. tests. Surely no responsibility or blame can be ascribed. With the introduction of awareness into the equation, however, the possibility for mastering one's
previously uncontrollable and damaging circumstances develops.
In the case of cancer-prone people, who usually maintain a suspicious attitude (at least on the unconscious level) more consistently
than others, the disease presents at the point in time when the body's
balancing apparatus is overwhelmed, resulting in toxicity at the
cellular level. Cancer cells are produced in this milieu, and repro-

duced at an alarming rate, since the system's defenses are degraded. The organism contracts and is unable to ward off or eliminate internal predators, e.g., bacteria, virus, poisons, cancer cells. What seems to be happening is, as the outer possibility for danger is constantly guarded against, the inner guard is compromised. Without its natural protection (of the immune system) a vicious toxic cycle (VTC), coined by Wallace, ensues.

Traditional medicine acknowledges the existence of the deranged cancer cells, as well as the organism's weakened state. Its strategy is to eliminate the expression (cancer) of the problem by surgery, chemotherapy or radiation. This symptom-oriented medicine often fails, since the root cause – faulty breath – has not been eliminated (or even identified). We must also note that aggressive, conventional methods tend to exacerbate the organism's contraction, first by the dreaded connotation that attends the diagnosis of cancer, second by the fear of the horrific medical procedures used, and finally by the shock that all surgery, chemotherapy, and radiation produces on the human system.

Gentler holistic remedies, on the other hand, address the problem at its origin, attempting to intervene on the VTC without further stressing the person. Unhealthy negative attitudes are substituted for by "imagery" of a positive nature. Strengthening the body through a detoxifying diet is a major goal, and deep breathing exercises that allow for elimination of unconscious conflict are initiated – all of which call for conscious patient participation.

Cancer patients repress and deny unpleasant effects, such as, depression, anxiety, guilt to a significantly higher degree than do the controlled subjects. Impaired emotional outlets are significantly pronounced in lung cancer patients. (Achterberg)

The strategy is to reawaken the innate tendency to healing through rebalancing all the systems of the person. Humor also has been publicly recognized as a healing tool, over the last decade, with publication of the book *Anatomy of An Illness Perceived by the Patient* (1979) in which Norman Cousin recounts how he recovered from cancer by watching old movies of the Three Stooges and laughing his head off.

For a serious psychosomatic disease such as cancer, the benefits to be derived from marijuana cannot be overstated:

1. The causal element of unconscious (repressed) pain can be

ferreted out.

2. The breath can be restored to fullness, thereby eliminating directly the built up toxicity and, at the same time, enjoining balance throughout the whole organism. A depressed system is a weakened system, and since it works holistically, marijuana gives strength where weakness exists, and expansion and relaxation where there is contraction and nervousness.

3. The more richly oxygenated blood that is in effect with marijuana can help to cleanse the poisons at the cellular level.

4. And a broader perspective through activation of the entire brain leads to positive feelings and thus eliminates the usual and debilitating attitudes so common in cancer – helplessness, depression, fear, resignation, and dread.

Application of Marijuana

Although today we know marijuana as a material for smoking, in ancient India and in the medical profession of the Western world, marijuana in liquid forms (known as bhang and tincture of cannabis, respectively) was most often utilized as a tonic and medicine. This method of application can easily eliminate any worry concerning carcinogenic substances that are suggested as a by-product of marijuana smoking. TINCTURE OF MARIJUANA is made from potent buds and over 100 "proof" alcohol. Measurements of 1 pint of alcohol to 1 ounce of bud are common. After two week of darkness, during which time the mixture is shaken on a daily basis, the plant material is strained from the alcohol (leaving the tincture.) It is administered in minute doses, because of its potency. If we look into the homeopathic Materia Medicas, tincture of cannabis is the common form of prescription.

The allegation that smoking marijuana may cause cancer and other lung problems may be baseless, however. In a Costa Rican study, it was found that chronic marijuana smokers who also smoked cigarettes, were less likely to develop cancer than those who didn't use marijuana. Since marijuana (smoking, as well as ingestion by other methods) dilates the alveoli, toxins are more easily eliminated with cannabis use regardless of its application. Nicotine, on the other hand, constricts the alveoli, so it is likely that the use of cannabis neutralizes, or even overwhelms the constriction, by its own tendency to dilation. Smoking marijuana, moreover, in cases of severe nausea, overrides the problem of taking medicine by mouth in patients who cannot "keep anything down" (Morgan, 1992).

As an aid for all psychosomatic disease, marijuana can benefit the participant, generally because of its health-restoring effects. Ironically, psychosomatic disease is fear expressed in its most potent form, while marijuana is feared because it will allow for the expression of fear in a more diffused and therefore less deadly fashion. The fear of marijuana also stems from its limitless potential for treating illness, in that both the pharmaceutical industry, as well as the medical monopoly, would lose billions of dollars, should marijuana become the non-drug of choice.

Marijuana is incredibly useful for chemotherapy patients, yet it is

---

A Recipe for Bhang* with Spices

- Milk (quart) and sugar (if desired).
- Dried Marihuana leaves and flowers, approx. 10 grams.
- Poppy seeds, pepper, dry ginger, caraway seeds, cloves, cinnamon, nutmeg (according to personal taste).

Boil vegetation in water for 5 minutes, mash/mush as it boils. Strain and discard the liquid. Take the residue (remaining plant material) and form into paste by mashing with back of spoon. Add milk (just enough to aid retention of ball-like consistency) Add whatever of other ingredients available (not the sugar or milk). Take ball and dissolve in a quart of milk – warming slowly over low flame. Strain milk and discard vegetation. Add a touch of sugar to milk. Color will be greenish. Refrigerate and drink when desired.

Mixture for 2 men in one day (or one woman for two days).

***Bhang**—Indian term for marijuana leaves and flowers dissolved in milk and taken as refreshing and health-giving drink. [*Hi-fat cow milk is the traditional extractor for Bhang, which was called SOMA in the ancient Vedic Scriptures — Editor*]
Recipe from pg. 480, *Memorandum to Indian Hemp Drugs Commission* 1969.

not allowed by the government, despite full knowledge of its extreme usefulness. Rumor has it, however, that physicians often inform their patients of marijuana's therapeutic effects and suggest that they obtain a dose on the illegal market. This is especially the case in the V.A. Hospitals, where chronic pain and boredom plague our former soldiers, and their long stay results in their doctors becoming their friends, and also in AIDS and cancer chemotheraphy patients.

Beginning in the 90s, in blatant disregard for the marijuana laws, a number of CBC's (Cannabis Buyers Clubs) formed to aid those with grave and terminal illness. These clubs actually distribute marijuana regularly, specifically to fill the void left by the government's refusal to recognize the medicinal benefits of marijuana. In the State of California, these clubs are working under the auspices of the 1996 Compassionate Use State Law. The Federal Government, however does not recognize their legality and on occasion, the DEA has raided these medical distribution centers, confiscating both medicine and property. Despite the laws, almost every major city has a CBC, and for the most part, little enforcement of the law has been forthcoming. Unfortunately, it seems reasonable to expect that government harassment will escalate as the extent of the benefits of marijuana become more widespread.

Because "chemo" poisons the system in its attempt to destroy cancer cells, the entire organism is in gross disequilibrium. Marijuana restabilizes the body very rapidly. The patient feels better, is no longer nauseous, and even experiences a desire to eat, which was unthinkable only moments ago. In fact, enhancement of appetite has a far greater meaning than just being able to eat. A person who feels well enough to take food is reaffirming life. The benefit may be seen only in the lunch taken, but the truth is that marijuana acts on the entire person, and not just the appetite, by restoring the depressed system to balance, which includes broadening the mental outlook. Recently scientific acknowledgment in the treatment of asthma, glaucoma, MS and AIDS-wasting syndrome has become publicized in keeping with the tides of change that cannot be resisted. (National Institute of Health , 9/22/97 - is calling for research into all aspects of marijuana therapy, following its recognition of the medical potential of cannabis.)

Marijuana: Limitless Remedial Action

Once we realize the general principle by which it affects the human system, marijuana potential uses are endless. This can be perhaps most dramatically documented with a list of recommended uses for marijuana, derived from *Ancient Uses of Marijuana* (McKenna, 1992). It was used as a remedy for malaria, beri-beri, constipation, rheumatic pain, absent-mindedness, female disorders, dysentery, leprosy, dandruff, headache, mania, venereal disease, whooping cough, earache, tuberculosis, snake bite, nodes/tumors, jaundice, glaucoma, asthma, muscular dystrophy, epilepsy, and excitability. It was used to quicken the mind, prolong life, improve judgement, lower fever, induce sleep, aid the bile, stimulate appetite, aid in childbirth, and better the voice. It was an antiphlegmatic, analgesic, mild sedative, tonic, anti-nauseant, and a digestive.

> In 19th century medicine, tincture of cannabis was used mostly as a sedative and antispasmodic for insomnia, migraine, epilepsy, excitability, childbirth, and menstrual discomfort. Interestingly enough, the medical reports from that time make little or no mention of psychoactive effects. People's expectations were different. Either they did not get high from it because they didn't expect to, or if they did, they paid it no attention and did not mention it to their doctors. (Weil, 1980, p. 95)

Modern medical recommendations of marijuana include using it as a painkiller, anti-asthmatic, anti-convulsant, anti-bratic, appetite promoter, anti-rheumatic, sedative, anti-diarrheal, anti-pyretic, anti-biotic, and anti-tumor (Mechoulam, 1990).

If the claims that marijuana is generally beneficial are true, it follows that its regular use may help prevent many illnesses. And it can be suggested that people otherwise predisposed to psychosomatic diseases (through mental/physical or lifestyle orientation), who have been regular marijuana users, will represent a much smaller percentage among the already afflicted than is true of the population at large. If this is the case, it would certainly rank marijuana among the most useful of preventive remedies. Whether a scientific study of this nature can be reasonably undertaken is another matter.

❖

DIVINE VISION
Joan Bello

In the cycle, unending of growth and pain
Toward the circle's bending to goodness again
The time returns to stand apart
It's come once more to stalk the heart

We have become a complex decay
A simple flower saves the day
The spark of the seed is holy and pure
The sight in the weed is offered for cure

As the spirit within the dove
Marijuana offers love
Be a temple, use the tools
Truth and flowers are God's jewels

Divine Vision personified
In a plant, simplified
With our reason nullified
By our laws crucified

TRANSACTION RECORD

T: CHAPTERS #770
  DALHOUSIE STN S.C.
  CALGARY   AB
ERMINAL: 00247208   OPERATOR: 00000407
ISA: 4500 6200 0009 8188   EXP 03/10

URCHASE:

$ 48.59

UTH. #:   006742   SWIPED
EFERENCE #:   2165   DATE: 01/08/15
ATCH #:   0860   TIME: 18:20:11
ARDHOLDER WILL PAY CARD ISSUER ABOVE
MOUNT PURSUANT TO CARDHOLDER AGREEMENT

IGNATURE: _____

    HAVE A NICE DAY ! BONNE JOURNEE !

Chapter 4 • Spiritual Benefits
The Third Dimension

It is relatively easy to demonstrate that marijuana is healthy for the body, since its physiological benefits can be tested objectively as well as subjectively by marijuana users. Psychological stability, although not quite so readily measurable, depends on an integration between the conscious and unconscious flow of ideas. Again, the effect of marijuana corresponds to the acceptable framework of healthy awareness. However, when we address the benefits of marijuana upon the inner fabric of humanness, we begin to tread on thin ice. Since this inner world cannot be seen or measured, the materialistic perspective tends to ignore its existence.

> In many societies, experimentation with growth beyond this level (of an effective ego) is not encouraged. In fact, if it involves an investment of energy that detracts even temporarily from one's material productivity, it may be actually discouraged. Investing time or energy into developing oneself beyond the ego level may be better understood or appreciated by a society where economic success and material possessions are not the major criteria by which one is judged. Experimentation with higher states of consciousness may be regarded with suspicion or considered wasteful nonsense. (Ajaya, 1977)

In the area of private values, marijuana may offer benefits beyond the personal ego, which reach the dimension referred to by mystics and saints as the ever-present "now." The experience addresses states of consciousness not common to the common man and resembles Maslow's "peak experience." Rather than being a concrete, stable reality, this realm approaches intuition and ecstasy; it apprehends an unusual connectedness with the whole of life. Daily existence becomes but an invisible script where what matters is the attitude by which one lives. In the world of thought and relationship, honesty and compassion are the prime motivators, while material gain and loss are secondary. This is really an ascension to religious values, not familiar or even welcomed within the context of modern society, but certainly containing great benefit for individual happiness. Our culture has become anti-religious. Our society is based on getting, not giving, and even though our words uphold virtue and love as worthy goals, hardly anyone even tries to live by such a philosophy. The regular use of marijuana, however, can often set the stage for receptivity to this higher knowledge or level of being.

Higher Consciousness

To ascend the ladder of consciousness, human beings need as much help as they can get. States of consciousness above the concerns of personal survival and power are neither necessary for human life, nor visible from ordinary states of mind. Because these states of consciousness threaten the power structure, all means to them are often outlawed. If we are not taught by some older, wiser person that deep and timeless perceptions really exist (or unless we ourselves fortuitously catch a glimpse of these subjective realities), we remain ignorant of their existence and thus are easily molded into the lower social goals of materialism, competition, and power. This less enlightened state of consciousness is expressed by a gnawing dissatisfaction unable to be eliminated. It is the dimension of perennial desire where, with each fulfillment of a goal/need/want, another void erapts. In Buddhism, it is the realm of nightmarish, insatiable hunger, which cannot be resolved unless, and until, the beinghood attains to a less self-centered level. Deep within each of us, an essential need for a higher meaning of life waits to be awakened. Because of its ability to unlock this yearning and allow us a glimpse of the deeper reality, marijuana is both feared by the establishment and loved by the user. Speaking about the personality change that some people undergo as a result of introduction to cannabis, Inglis (1975) says that it

...does not intoxicate...is not addictive...But (it) confronts society with an issue that it has been unwilling to face. People may need (this) not in (its) own right, but as a preliminary to restoration of the link, largely lost, between man's (and woman's) consciousness, and all that lies beyond it. The personality change may be for their benefit! (p. 229)

Quoting from the La Dain Committee, he continues:

The positive values people find in the...experience bear a striking similarity to traditional religious values, including the concern with soul, or inner self. The Spirit of renunciation, the emphasis on openness and the closely-knit community are part of it, but this is definitely a sense of identification with something larger, something to which one belongs as part of the human race. (p. 229)

It is mainly because spiritual values are abandoned during eras of materialism that marijuana is banned today. And, ironically, it is because these values are so absent in the modern culture that the marijuana experience is so ardently sought.

> Despite all the pressures brought against it, cannabis use rose until today (it) may well be America's single largest agricultural product...the innate drive to restore the psychological balance typifying (a) partnership society, once it finds a suitable vehicle, is not easily deterred. (McKenna, 1992, p. 165)

The regular use of marijuana is a sane attempt at adaptation that occurs spontaneously among certain marginal members of a group. Without an "evolutionary leap" in human priorities, the danger of extinction is real. Evolution for human beings is toward an expansion of consciousness, or cooperation, in response to present-day alienation.

The Science of Vibration

Thousands of years ago, in a non-hostile climate, known today as the cradle of civilization, marijuana was used extensively. Out from this Eden-like existence, a profound spiritual cosmology developed. "The Science of Vibration" is as valid today as it was then, but progression to our modern lifestyle (and away from inner values) excluded interest in it. Only in the last few decades has the industrialized world paid it any serious attention. Perhaps investigation into the higher human values could not surface in the industrial West until all imaginable physical, psychological, and social dysfunction reached dangerous proportions. Perhaps the further a culture falls from recognizing the realm of the sacred, the more need exists for it to do so. Whatever the explanation, whatever the impetus, there can be no doubt of the interest that exists today concerning higher consciousness. This interest represents a dynamic tension pulling against the material ethic, for which marijuana has served as an abiding ally.

In the Eastern sciences, the vibrational makeup of creation is evidenced not only in the cosmos, but also through the human form, which is recognized as a miniature representation of the universe. Whatever principles apply to the macrocosm and its processes apply equally to the functioning of human life. With this logic, and with extensive personal experimentation, it has been discovered that the human body has a containment of powerful energy polarized along the spinal column, divided into a dynamic negative charge (at the base of the spine) and a static positive charge (at the crown of the head) – very much in keeping with the magnetism and repulsion of electromagnetic fields. Only a minuscule percentage of the total charge is used to maintain the organism, leaving a vast surplus of potential energy untapped. To trigger this dormant energy – to transverse the entire spinal pathway – stands as the highest goal of life in Eastern philosophy. With such a release, likened to the "nuclear energy of the psycho/physical system" (Saraswati, 1984), the human being is said to fulfill his/her potential.

The ascent of this charge follows the vertical column within the spine in much the same way that electricity is born along a lightening rod. As it flows upward, with the speed of light, it passes through intricate electromagnetic centers of the body that result from congested intersections of major nerves and organs. These centers are called "chakras" in the East, and they correspond to modes of behavior or levels of understanding. Although they are not visible, the chakras' fields of energetic congestion are measurable and, in the West, are just beginning to be investigated. Weil and Rosen (1983), pioneers of Western Holistic Medicine, explain it this way:

> Potential circuits exist for conducting unconscious impulses upward, as anyone knows who is aware of his daydreams and intuitions. The sealing of these channels from above forces unbalanced, unconscious energies down the autonomic nerves to produce negative physical effects...If we never learn to open these channels by disengaging our minds from ordinary consciousness, we condemn ourselves to sickness. (p. 63)

As we have seen, marijuana's effect on the brain, although surely not as dramatic as total release of this contained psychonuclear charge, offers a similar, if toned down, replication. It lends a taste to this intuitive faculty, and for that reason, along with meditation and yoga, marijuana has been consistently employed by Eastern spiritual practices.

> When the right hemisphere of the brain is especially stimulated, latent intuitive powers of extrasensory perceptions, such as clairvoyance, telepathy begin to be unfolded. (Saraswati, 1984)

Eastern Yogic thinking has long recognized the two modes of the mind:

> The brain has two major modes or systems, which must work together and be harmonized if we are not to lose the essentials of our human existence. Unfortunately, few of us are really balanced and most of us, especially men, tend towards the purely external, materialistic and technological...side rather than the subtle, intuitive, feeling side...Most of us fluctuate, according to our inner biological rhythms, moving from left to right brain, right to left nostril, active to receptive mode...From the yogic point of view, this rhythmic, or in the case of disease, arrhythmic swing, indicates that we are unbalanced and that one mode, one side of our nature is constantly becoming predominant. We rarely experience the more desirable state in which both sides become equal and balanced. According to yoga, when both the sad [left] and happy [right] hemispheres are balanced for a certain length of time, a new state arises which unites logic and intuition, transforms our emotions and enables us to power a greater range of neurological activity. (ibid, p. 365-367)

The Christian mystic de Chardin, explaining this same process, says "physical energy must be mastered and grounded for spiritual energy to move, because physical energy transforms the spirit" (Ferguson, 1973). Within the deep recesses of human understanding, the intuitive faculty steers its course. For many who are in touch with this sixth sense, the realm of the spirit is supreme. Anything that demonstrates a possibility for psycho/spiritual uplifting is known to be sacred. Marijuana is so recognized and revered. "Bhang brings union with the Divine Spirit." (Indian Hemp Drugs Commission, 1969, p. 491)

Evolution of a person is demarcated by stages in all esoteric teachings. "The Theory of Vibration" is a seven-fold ascension that originates in the lowest human emotion of instinctive survival, situated at the base of the spine, and rises to the highest experience of pure awareness, above the crown of the head (as a halo). Seven is a mystical number in all esoteric religions, as it represents the stages of possible human evolution. Its meaning has, for the most part, been forgotten. In this model, each level of psycho-spiritual evolvement has a corresponding energetic density and a geographical site ("chakra") in the body. Every person displays a certain attitude, a predominant way of perceiving both inner and outer worlds, and also a type of action depending upon his/her stage of evolution. At the lower levels, which Freud studied extensively, there is an animal-like nature ("id") that is concerned solely with personal survival. This is an accurate account of the qualities of the low, second "level" (chakra) attitude. Freud's investigations were not concerned with demonstrating the evolutionary possibilities of humanness. His patients were limited by their extreme pathologies, and his own intellectual model did not envision development beyond an ego driven, always, only by primal desire.

Conscience

With marijuana, we uncover the unconscious creative understanding that is usually hidden, since as we have seen, right brain energizing brings an expansion in awareness (or witness). It is not the right hemisphere's increased activity alone that expands awareness. It is the balancing mode that is born with additional activity in the right hemisphere – responsible for heightened consciousness.

Balance is the stage of human development from which the "objective witness" is born. It implies harmony in all areas of life, so that no distraction or restriction interferes with growth toward the fullness of human potential. The difference between consciousness with a 'witness' and ordinary consciousness is none other than the difference between operating with a conscience or without one. In ordinary life, we are all bound by Freud's superego, which maintains our behavior according to the social ideals we have been taught. This is the (internalized) repressive element of civilization, which restrains our animal natures from actions considered harmful to society, our church, our parents, and our peers. Without it, normal social life could not continue.

The Ten Commandments were presented to a social group that no longer functioned conscientiously and therefore needed mandatory direction. Within the deeper levels of human nature, however, an objective, timeless, universal sense of right and wrong exists. This is conscience. Unfortunately, the rules of our world are far removed from this inherent, eternal, inner understanding of right action. Our inner world can know, but our imbalanced way of life does not allow for its fruition. From a vibrational perspective this can be understood as a lack of energy, excessive resistance, or low charge – all due to disharmony. Through balance, with time and interest, marijuana can enliven the "Center of Knowing." In the Theory of Vibration, this is the sixth level of development known as the "Knowledge Center." What we refer to as the sixth sense, or intuition, derives from this esoteric symbol, which very often is depicted as a third eye, located at the midbrow:

> ...where the mind perceives knowledge directly, via a sixth or intuitive sense, which comes into operation as the sixth (knowledge) chakra awakens....where one becomes the detached observer of all events, including those within the body and mind...often, the experience one has when awakening takes place in the Ajna Chakra (Knowledge Center) is similar to that induced by marijuana. (Saraswati, 1984, p. 138)

Jesus Christ referred to this very same awakening that is evidenced within the body: "If therefore thine eye be single, thy whole body shall be full of light." (Matthew 6:22)

Consequences of Conscience

As we have seen, many an argument against marijuana refers to the non-competitive nature it engenders. During the Vietnam War, one of the major problems of our soldiers was their inability to accept the brutality of their own actions. Our young men encountered marijuana at every turn in Asia (the Vietnam War was the beginning of marijuana use in this country, since it was the first time a status and educational cross-section of America was exposed to it), and their reaction was often not in keeping with the insensitivity necessary for war. Their conscience bothered them. Gaining higher values, such as compassion, cooperation, and consideration, is a function of balance and a threat to a militaristic society. If we all became aware of our conscience, who would be left to maintain the indifference of the social order? The more we uncover the spiritual element in our natures, the more sensitive we become. Scrooge had no conscience until he experienced the spirit. He was surely happier and healthier after his vision, but not wealthier, for his conscience dictated that he share. His new-felt sensitivity did not result from rules, fear, or his superego. It overflowed joyfully as an expression of his higher state of being.

Marijuana's contribution to the developing spirit is cumulative.

As bodily tensions are reduced, mental fears dissolve, clearing the way to greater insight. But, until the direct effect (physical balance) of marijuana on the body and the attendant side effect (high) of marijuana in the mind become familiar, the alterations themselves remain the focus of interest. The "getting high" is the end in itself, rather than the understanding and insight that accrues as the changed set becomes more common. People who try marijuana and reject it do so usually because they feel uncomfortable and confused in the altered, fuller consciousness. Instead of life being safely framed by the rigidity of the societal dogma, the world becomes unfamiliarly bigger, brighter, fuller, yet less manageable, more unpredictable and full of mystery. A mind that has been bound and accustomed to a low charge or a setting without light very often finds the expansiveness of reality too highly energized. The light can be blinding and disorienting. Over time, and with regular intake, when these higher states of seeing are no longer the focal point of attention, a restructuring of values may emerge.

Holistic Framework of Body/Mind/Spirit

In the ancient philosophies there was no division between medicine, psychology, or religion. Today's conventional disciplines split the body from the mind and only grudgingly acknowledge the possibility of spirit. The medical doctor administers to the body, the psychologist to the mind, and the priest to the somewhat elusive notion of the spirit. In contrast with these divisions, holistic health (integrating psychology, medicine, and spiritual counseling) has gained a foothold in prevailing attitudes. By tapping the wisdom of ancient civilizations, and demonstrating its validity through modern techniques, a new potential for understanding human life is available to this time period. Less restriction, more tolerance, less fear, more compassion, all qualities of higher consciousness, are functions of long-term marijuana use.

The three human centers of body/mind/spirit were realized, studied, and suppressed many times over the course of human existence. Evidence supports the notion that esoteric knowledge arrived at the same conclusion from all diverse areas (Sufis, Hopis, Cabalists) of human habitation around the world, only to be lost amid the cyclical ebb and flow of various cultural upheavals. *The Gnostic Gospels*, long denied existence by the Church Fathers, uphold a less material-bound ethic, closer to the deeper values of true religion. These Gospels are spiritually focused and speak to the higher nature, calling for introspection and subjective interpretation of private experiences, instead of reliance on an outer authority such as the institution of church. Understandably they represented a threat to organized religion. "Their existence was simply denied until the last decade when the truth was finally publicized," (*The Gnostic Gospels*, Pagels). The Catholic Church still denies their validity.

The timeless, higher values have been submerged over the entire gamut of what is termed "modern" history (600 years or so). In their place, religious institutions set forth regulations that serve the organizations, and the pleasure of fellowship, but hold little possibility for personal experiences of joy. The esoteric kernel of merger with the sublime has been lost and, with it, the methods to attain to full understanding. Yet, by definition, true religion strives to increase wisdom and compassion. That is why, to many, the marijuana experience is religious. It allows for a more meaningful assessment of the whole of life when unstable elements of the personality are resolved.

All experience, say the mystics, is but one piece of an infinite puzzle. Science continually discovers a piece at a time. This modern practice overlooks the forest for the trees. The cooperation of body/ mind/spirit is the ultimate holistic framework of human potential, but generally escapes our modern, materialistic minds. Marijuana, an ancient plant used for thousands of years, throughout ancient civilizations to benefit this integration, is being used today for this very same reason by persons who love the effect it has on them and their lives, without exactly understanding its operation. Hopefully, we have lessened that ignorance.

The Question of Soul

The mechanical models of biology had a strong influence on medicine (and all the social sciences) which has come to regard the human body as a machine. Scientists treat matter as dead and completely separate from themselves. —Capra

Modern psychology has sought to disassociate from religious beliefs...to show itself to have a scientific attitude. —Ajaya

In order to present my holistic ideas, I almost fell into the "scientific" trap. It once seemed that only by a thoroughly objective analysis of the way marijuana affects the body and the mind might I be able to impart the extensive benefits of this ancient plant. For example, five years ago, a major publisher of books on marijuana offered to purchase this book when it was just a manuscript, providing I would agree to drop the Spiritual Benefits of Marijuana chapter, which he explained was apt to be a "turn off" to the secular mainstream. I had to decline this early offer to publish my findings, because I had not espoused or even addressed nearly as much as I believe concerning the mysterious Divinity that abides within marijuana. I could not agree to drop the spiritual segment and still remain true to my purpose in writing this book.

Above all else, I yearn to display the wonderful and long forgotten healing qualities of marijuana to everyone, from politicians to doctors, from substance abuse counselors to all stressed and sick people, because I believe that the immortal soul orchestrates our every turn and explains the workings of the body and mind. My entire premise is based on this: that directing all human functions is the individual, indivisible, immortal soul.

There is an ancient Hindu narrative that is well-known to students of Yogic Science. It clarifies the posture responsible for the East's seemingly limitless knowledge of the labyrinthine workings of the Universe (the human organism included) – while at the same time uncovering the disparity between the reductionistic methodology of Western Materialism.

"There is a River. It flows with observable rhythm, in harmony with the Celestial Lights. The Eastern student notices this fact, in quietude with absorbed and one-pointed interest. The river's existence is sustenance to all flora and fauna in its path – all of which the student scrutinizes and registers to memory. The tributaries of the river give life to the crops and allow for the continuation of the (past and present) groupings of civilization, as well as all domesticated and wild animals, all flowers and edible vegetation. This the student studies, learning how and when the river ebbs and flows, down to its most minuscule cause and effect (without any self-serving motive to alter or control this natural process). Because of none other than innate curiousity to understand the Cause of all that is Created, the seeker begins his (her) investigation. The search is slow, encompassing the student's entire thrust and takes the seeker to ever higher levels up the mountain, where everything becomes finer, purer, or in other words more simple and predictable.

With each ascension to the next higher plateau, less and less baggage may be carried. Less dense forms of eating, thinking and breathing are natural to this learning process which allows for subjective perceptions to become more lucid since less diversions abound as the climb contnues to The Single Source of All.

After endless study, always of an experiential nature, the serious seeker reaches to the top of the mountain – from which springs the river in endless profusion. At this point – is the attainment of yogic satisfaction – at the Third Eye – where the individual soul knows itself in direct relationship to the Mystery (since the body and mind have been purified and are no longer hindrances – the goal of yoga).

Atop the rock, sits a Western scientist, having arrived (typically) by helicopter, without benefit of noticing any of the precise workings of the eternal flow. The Westerner has much baggage in the way of apparel and apparatus to aid in breathing the thin air, not having gotten accustomed to such fine oxygen over time (electronic devices and modern communication tools as well – in abundance). The scientist plans to tap the source for profit. S/he notices the yogi(ni), who has shed almost all baggage, attire, and even food stuff, sitting in idle and blissful oblivion.

The scientist asks the typical question that mechanically springs to a grasping, information-filled head: 'Why and How does the water flow?'

The yogi(ni) departs from silence – astonished that such a question is being asked. S/he answers: 'Thou are That' (which is of contemptible disinterest to the scientist).

This story has many variations. Sometimes it is longer or shorter. It serves the listener to realize that the Source is mysterious, to be realized and appreciated as the Blessedness it is – not to be challenged or changed. This "knowing" is the level of being compatible with Marijuana as a Sacrament, where the individual soul is intuitively aided in realization of the Divine by the inherent vibration within the plant. It is said that at the sixth ("ajna") chakra, one recognizes unitary consciousness from the perspective of the pureness of the unencumbered soul.

The ultimate state of consciousness in the Eastern understanding of the human possibility for evolution is to realize one's own true nature as identical with that illimitable, immortal consciousness – Existence, Knowledge, and Bliss ("sat, chit, ananda"). By the grace of the Mystery and through the receptiveness of no division ("advaita"), and absolutely not under the control of the seeker, the aspirant's consciousness enters the realm of Unity – joining with the ocean of Unitary Consciousness as all separate waves ultimately do so that the "observer and observed are one" (Krishnamurti, 1971).

And the moral of the story is: The precision and predictability of the workings of the human organism – physical, psychological, and spiritual aspects of our nature, just as in the boundless universe, can be observed and understood, with patience, interest and lack of prejudice to an amazing degree of depth, which the Western mind has rarely comprehended. The magnetism of the desire for knowledge, alone, will sustain the seeker, only if all preconceived notions and self-serving motives are considered expendable. This is the purification process of yogic practices. All aids to such purification are valid. Once a method for un-coupling from our baggage of conditioning and possessions is discovered, IT is unquestionably to be embraced and even worshipped. This is the teaching of the Tantra, the most profound body of religious thought of all Eastern discipline. The HEMP is one such Holy Aid. The Buddha is often depicted in naked meditation with but one hemp seed for nurturance.

In truth, it is the soul that is impacted most prominently with marijuana, and all the intricate, measurable, observable, and subjective bodily and mental effects that I have explained so carefully (and so carefully admitting of no such directorship) are secondary to the conscious impact and omniscience of the Source that may be imparted to the true seeker by the mystery within the marijuana plant.

I think if I had to explain – in the fewest words possible – exactly what it is that marijuana does, I would have to steal these words from Guy Mount: "It lifts the spirit." That idea so aptly describes the benefits of marijuana whether viewed from a physical, psychological, or spiritual perspective. If by admitting there is a soul within everything alive on this planet, and that everything, including the planet itself is alive, I "turn off" the secular, scientifically-bound mindset of anyone – let it be!

TO SAVE YOUR SOUL
Joan Bello

Do you smoke the weed
Do you know its treasure
Do you save the seed
To grow yourself more pleasure

Then I can talk to you
And you to me
For you are one of those
Who always wants to see

That this life without a goal
Makes you want to cry
So you smoke—To save your soul
And help your spirit fly

PROPOSITION 215: MEDICAL MARIJUANA
Passed into law by a vote of the People of California
November 5, 1996 • Yes: 55% • No: 45%

SUMMARY OF THE COMPASSIONATE USE ACT OF 1996

Exempts from criminal laws patients and defined caregivers who possess or cultivate marijuana for medical treatment recommended by a physician. Provides physicians who recommend use shall not be punished. Fiscal Impact: Probably no significant fiscal impact on state and local governments.

* Exempts patients and defined caregivers who possess or cultivate marijuana for medical treatment recommended by a physician from criminal laws which otherwise prohibit possession or cultivation of marijuana.

* Provides physicians who recommend use of marijuana for medical treatment shall not be punished or denied any right or privilege.

* Declares that measure not be construed to supersede prohibitions of conduct endangering others or to condone diversion of marijuana for nonmedical purposes.

* Contains severability clause.

TEXT OF COMPASSIONATE USE ACT OF 1996

Section 1. Section 11362.5 is added to the Health and Safety Code, to read:

11362.5. (a) This section shall be known and may be cited as the Compassionate Use Act of 1996.

(b) (l) The people of the State of California hereby find and declare that the purposes of the Compassionate Use Act of 1996 are as follows:

(A) To ensure that seriously ill Californians have the right to obtain and use marijuana for medical purposes where that medical use is deemed appropriate and has been recommended by a physician who has determined that the person's health would benefit from the use of marijuana in the treatment of cancer, anorexia, AIDS, chronic pain, spasticity, glaucoma, arthritis, migraine, or any other illness for which marijuana provides relief.

B) To ensure that patients and their primary caregivers who obtain and use marijuana for medical purposes upon the recommendation of a physician are not subject to criminal prosecution or sanction.

(C) To encourage the federal and state governments to implement a plan to provide for the safe and affordable distribution of marijuana to all patients in medical need of marijuana.

(2) Nothing in this act shall be construed to supersede legislation prohibiting persons from engaging in conduct that endangers others, nor to condone the diversion of marijuana for nonmedical purposes.

(c) Notwithstanding any other provision of law, no physician in this state shall be punished, or denied any right or privilege, for having recommended marijuana to a patient for medical purposes.

(d) Section 11357, relating to the possession of marijuana, and

Section 11358, relating to the cultivation of marijuana, shall not apply to a patient, or to a patient's primary caregiver, who possesses or cultivates marijuana for the personal medical purposes of the patient upon the written or oral recommendation or approval of a physician.

(e) For the purposes of this section, "primary caregiver" means the individual designated by the person exempted under this act who has consistently assumed responsibility for the housing, health, or safety of that person.

Sec. 2. If any provision of this measure or the application thereof to any person or circumstance is held invalid, that invalidity shall not affect other provisions or applications of the measure which can be given effect without the invalid provision or application, and to this end the provisions of this measure are severable.

Chapter 5 • Marijuana Therapy
The Eastern Understanding

I was very lucky to receive a rigorous and non-conventional Graduate course of study, under the direct guidance of an advanced yogi, specifically to prepare me "to be a bridge" between the ancient Eastern wisdom and modern Western science. I never knew how that awesome mission would unfold, but with my research with cannabis over the last decade I have learned.

The teaching professors for the Graduate course were licensed M.D.s and Ph.D.s from highly-acclaimed universities: Harvard/ Duke/Chicago/Buffalo, or equally prestigious Oriental schools. The students, as well as the American faculty, had all gravitated to the precise and extensive knowledge of the immense body of thought, known as Indian Philosophy, out of a deep-felt need that Western "science" could not satisfy. Originally I came to the facility because it was instrumental in curing my son of his grande mal epilepsy. When a Master's in Science Degree at the Institute was offered, there was no doubt in my mind that it was the training I needed.

The Indian tradition spans 5000 years of accumulated knowledge, under which the sciences of religion, psychology, and medicine are interdependent and completely compatible; its depth of understanding flew in the face of modern belief systems and was vastly superior to them. In Ayurveda (traditional Indian medicine) the physician is responsible for guiding the student to "full spiritual integration with the universe" – considered the only worthy goal of human existence. This requires, first of all, health of body and mind, which is understood as a progressive, intentional purification process. Throughout the history of India, the cannabis plant has played a major role for: growth in the spirit, peace of the mind, and medicine for the body, not to mention the myriad industrial uses which it served for millennia.

During my formal studies, Marijuana Therapy was not discussed at all owing to its taboo in modern American culture. But the extensive private research library was full with treasures of Eastern medical tomes and "Oriental Studies' Journals" which gave cannabis its rightful place in health and attainment to higher consciousness. This library was where I spent most of my time during the five years that I was a student. I began collecting and studying these books and journals voraciously. Occasionally, I took courage to question the doctors about the effect of the herb. It always elicited the same response: *"a unique sedative-stimulant."* The subject would end in an awkward silence that I was understandably afraid to pursue.

Since, in the Eastern framework, a balanced Autonomic Nervous system is health, as well as a prerequisite for realization of the highest truth, all practice (diet/yoga/meditation) was toward that end. The student body was very small and we were painstakingly trained as scientific experimenters, acknowledging and recording our experiential reactions, as well as the objective, more-easily-measured responses of the body. Subjective reality is without merit in the West, but the Eastern tradition considers it of utmost importance. Through all of the experimentation, the goal was to become totally alert, while completely at ease, a state that can be translated as a dynamic tension between excitation and relaxation or *"sedation/stimulation."* All my free time was spent researching the unique hemp plant which had become very important in my life. I was not introduced to it until I was nearly 30 years old. Perhaps this fact played a major role in the impelling impact it had on my consciousness. Perhaps there is a more esoteric explanation for my one-pointed interest. Whatever the reason – I was avidly curious to prove what I suspected: that marijuana stabilizes the unconscious, automatic reactions of the human organism. Most of my fellow students acknowledged that cannabis enhanced mental faculties and physical well-being, but I was alone in my zealousness to learn just how it worked.

From one of our more outspoken American professors, the mystery of the ecstacy gained with LSD was revealed as a "flooding of both sides of the ANS." He explained that it mimicked the orgasmic reaction and was similar to the state attained in the highest consciousness, where the bliss of life is manifest. From that gem of information, in conjunction with the Science of Breath, and the accumulation of my research, I began to piece together the unrealized balancing ability of marijuana on the ANS. There was also one other important factor that spurred me on in my research – my son's epilepsy.

Although they were careful never to proselytize the benefits of marijuana, the actions of holistic practitioners belied their silence. About 10 years before I became a student, my 11-year-old son was a patient at the Homeopathic Clinic. I took him there in a desperate attempt to find a cure for his progressively worsening epilepsy. Conventional medical treatment had not helped him (despite prescriptions of increasingly aggressive drugs). Being the mischievous child that he was, during his weekly out-patient visit, my young son would confide to his assigned doctors (there were three of them) that he smoked marijuana regularly and with my knowledge. I would sit quietly in the corner, trying to melt into the walls, but unable to admonish him, because I knew that holistic treatment required total honesty. The oddest part of the story is that not one of his doctors ever admonished him either. At the end of the weekly hour-long session, they would always remind us both: "no potato chips, no meat, and no antibiotic medication." Whenever he became ill, my husband and I would take him to the clinic for a "remedy" that usually worked – seemingly miraculously – in 24 hours. After six months of intensive holistic health practice with appropriate homeopathic treatment, my son was cured. That was 20 years ago.

Needless to say, I am forever grateful. His cure, along with the silent sanctioning of his use of regular cannabis, is the reason I became a student of Eastern Science and took on the awesome responsibility of serving as a bridge between the East and the West. With the completion of this work, I feel somewhat relieved of that mandate but I also know that my work in the field of Marijuana Therapy is not yet finished.

Viewpoints: East and West

In defining Holistic Health, *holistic* refers to the whole person – body, mind and spirit, and *health* is the harmonious interplay of these three levels of humanness. Whereas lost equilibrium manifests itself as disease!

Modern Western medicine would not question anything so obviously true, but neither would it be interested in it. First of all, a three-dimensional model of human life is beyond the framework of 20th century science which focuses almost exclusively on the physical, as a natural consequence of cultural materialism. In such an agenda, only what we can own, see, taste and touch is valued. The underlying cause for the physical manifestation is not considered. The notion that automatic body processes are coordinated by an invisible component is meaningless from such an "objective scientific" approach. Although the medical profession never denies the existence of a life force, no serious study of the magnitude of its input on health is addressed. The Eastern understanding that full health implies interconnected harmony of the physical, mental, and spiritual realms of human life manifesting as a dynamic balance of the Autonomic Nervous System has not been studied in the West, nor is there any reason to believe it will be in the near future. It would require a total revolution both philosophically and economically, since conventional therapy today is so heavily invested (on all levels) in an aggressive path of research for external management of disease symptoms. In the Western model, the doctor is the authority and the patient follows instructions. Illness is inflicted on the afflicted from the outside. Whereas, in the ancient holistic Ayurvedic tradition, illness is an expression of disharmony from within. Treatment is a determined and joint investigation of the root cause by both the student and the teacher, an endeavor which will ultimately result in a purposeful change in behavior.

The sad fact is that disciplined, self-regulated change is not part of the educational repertoire of our culture. A secular society, disinterested in the underlying nature of reality and correspondingly indifferent to the possibility that regulating behavior can help prevent disease, cannot embrace the basic tenets of Holistic Health.

> *As it is not proper to try to cure the eyes without the head,*
> *nor the head without the body, so neither is it proper to cure*
> *the body without the soul, and this is the reason why so·*
> *many diseases escape (Greek) physicians who are ignorant*
> *of the whole. —Plato*

From that timeless 3000 year old quote, we can see that the problem of lifestyle causing sickness has not really changed, and that, in general, the 'physicians' outlook has maintained its narrow focus.

> *So you think our medicine is primitive?*
> *That's the wrong word. It isn't primitive. It's fifty per cent*

> *terrific and fifty per cent nonexistent. Marvelous antibiot-*
> *ics – but absolutely no methods for increasing resistance,*
> *so that antibiotics won't be necessary. Fantastic opera-*
> *tions – but when it comes to teaching people the way of*
> *going through life without having to be chopped up –*
> *absolutely nothing. Apart from sewage systems and syn-*
> *thetic vitamins, you don't seem to do anything at all about*
> *prevention and yet you have a proverb: "prevention is*
> *better than cure." —Aldous Huxley*

In those areas where technique and machines can x-ray a fracture, help the precision of operations, and, maybe soon, perform operations with greater precision than even the best of surgeons, and including all the incredible emergency medical procedures that have been developed in the last century, Western Medicine has made boundless and unequalled strides. In the area of internal disharmony (the natural consequence of habits that are unhealthy but nevertheless widespread), the ancient understanding is undeniably superior.

Historical Uses for Cannabis

Down through the centuries in nearly all kinds of cultures throughout the entire world, cannabis has been acknowledged as a unique and invaluable regulator, if not a "gift of the gods."

From the *Medicinal Plants of India & Pakistan*, cannabis is listed as "bhang, charas, ganja, hashish, subzee, vijaya." Every part of this wondrous plant was used for numerous ailments.

The leaves are sedative, anodyne, narcotic, antispasmodic, diuretic, digestive and astringent; as a sedative and anodyne they are given in doses of 40 grains; in dysentery and diarrhoea half a drachm of the dried leaves are given with sugar and black pepper; the leaves are administered to induce sleep where opium cannot be used; they are also used in tetanus and dysmenorrhoea. A paste of the fresh leaves is used to resolve tumors; their juice removes dandruff and head lice; their powder is a useful dressing for wounds and sores; a poultice of the leaves is applied to the eyes in ophthalmia and other diseases, and to piles.

The preparation made from specially dried leaves and flowers, known as bhang or hashish, is given in dyspepsia, gonorrhea and bowel complaints and as appetizer and nervine stimulant.

The dried pistillate flowering tops, coated with a resinous exudation are known as ganja; the smoke from burning ganga is swallowed as an antidote to poisoning. The smoke is passed through the rectum for relief of strangulated hernia and gripping pains of dysentery. It is given in one-fourth to two grain doses.

This latter, anal remedy, leaves us to wonder about the other receptors, not connected with the hypothalamus, that might exist on the surfaces of, and within internal organs of, our bodies. Receptors recently discovered and published in scientific journals only touch on this idea.)

It is locally used to relieve pain in itching skin diseases.

Charas, the resinous exudation that collects on the leaves....is of great value in malarial and periodic headaches, migraine, acute mania, insanity, delirium, whooping cough...asthma, anaemia of brain, nervous vomiting, tetanus, convulsions, nervous exhaustion and dysuria; it is also used as an anaesthetic in dysmenorrhea, as an appetizer, as an aphrodisiac...in eczema, neuralgia, severe pains, etc; it is usually given in one sixth to one fourth grain doses.

The seeds are used in infusion for gonorrhea.

The author J.F. Datur makes a statement at the beginning of his book that, unfortunately, prognosticates exactly what has occurred: "with the advancement of pharmaceutical researches, there is an increasing exploitation of our resources" (1962). But we are uncovering the ancient truths again – that natural marijuana is a miraculous medicine.

And from the *Materia Medica* by Ruddock in homeopathic treatment, cannabis is recommended:

...for difficulty of urinating, and menstrual headache is sometimes greatly helped; for opacity of cataract and specks on the cornea. For constipation. In humid asthma, and the effects of alcoholic intoxication.

The following studies are based on just a tiny sampling of the already existant Western-style documentation available and waiting to be integrated with the measured effects of marijuana that reveal why this primal earth medicine has enjoyed such ubiquitous, ancient and long-standing recognition. Its rediscovery by the modern world is an event whose time is at hand. Hopefully the following research will help to bridge the gap between the traditions of intuitive realization and the science of objective knowledge.

The Herb and Epilepsy

For the first 30 years of my life, my rebellious nature would occasionally show itself, but for the most part, I was mainstream mediocrity – all the way. Then, when I found the herb, all the conditioning of socialization, law-abidingness, organized religion, and social correctness lost its importance. Simplicity and honesty and kindness became ultra-significant, which of course changed everything. I entered the realm of altered consciousness which felt magically religious. I was Alice looking out and looking in – all at once, and I recognized this feeling in the pit of my being. It was eternally familiar, but absolutely new.

I'm a serious person by nature, that didn't change. Getting high let me understand that there is always profound meaning behind the script. Most importantly, it let me be who I had always known I was, deep down, like a "conversion." It was that dramatic! I acted almost immediately to share this wonder with my son. He was six and had suffered from seizures for the past four years.

Back in the early 70's no one talked about the medicinal value of marijuana, but I knew that it would help Steven. It took a long time, nearly 5 years. He gave up phenobarb, went to a Swami, was treated with homeopathy, and always used pot. Slowly his hyperactivity subsided. Then when he was 11, his epilepsy disappeared. I'm sure the Swami and the homeopathic physicians were instrumental in his cure. I'm just as sure that daily marijuana helped to set the needed tone of receptivity.

Steven is 31 now, works in the high-pressure mortgage business, still has an intense character, but never has a seizure. Like millions of people in America, he uses marijuana regularly – just like my other sons.

Because of our love and trust in this holy herb, we have suffered religious persecution at the hands of the state. My husband served time in prison. I spent time in jail. Our family savings went to the Criminal Injustice System. Our home has been uprooted. From afar it seems we have lost so much of value. But we keep the magic.

Alcoholism

As a Drug and Alcohol Counselor, I witnessed firsthand the devastating effects of alcoholism. Unfortunately, throughout the three years that I was employed by a county agency, I can report very few long-term success stories, and my colleagues would be in total agreement. There were actually only two. Both were mothers who had lost custody of their young children owing to their alcoholism. I followed their progress after the protracted battle with social services to regain their children and was happy to find out that, even after four years, they were both free from alcohol. But their stories are the exception. Even for those clients who were entirely sober for years, either because of imprisonment or threat of imprisonment, as soon as the legal reason was gone, so was their sobriety.

The psychological problems that cause alcoholism are unconscious fears and feelings of despondency which understandably cause a strong urge to numb the mental anguish and its attendant physical nervousness. Alcohol does this quickly, surely, legally, and lethally. Once the addiction is ingrained, only an overwhelming motivation is enough reason to endure the extreme discomfort of withdrawal.

"Alcoholics Anonymous" is the only treatment modality that conventional medicine acknowledges. It works for only a select number of alcoholics who: 1) first and foremost, desperately want to attain sobriety; 2) are able to face at least some of their hidden agenda; 3) are not adverse to the religious basis and bias of AA; and 4) who can substitute coffee, confession, and camaraderie in place of alcohol. But the sad fact is that most alcoholics never really seriously try to stop drinking until it's too late and the diagnosis is grave.

After three years with the county, I went into private practice. I was no longer limited by legal restrictions or fear of losing my job, and so I could put into practice what I had learned as a student of Holistic Health and Eastern Studies:

1. Self-Awareness and Self-Discipline are of utmost importance when regulating one's own behavior.

2. Don't bite off more than you can chew.

3. To break a bad habit, a good one must be substituted.

These three tenets are really in contradiction to the ideology underlying the AA model, which teaches alcoholics to relinquish control to a power greater than oneself and to stop all drinking immediately. In yogic psychology, we begin with gradual substitution of healthy habits. Self-awareness reigns supreme, and through it one regains control of the ability to direct one's own actions. Moderation is the message, so that total abstinence is not expected at first (as in the AA model) because it is so difficult, and ultimately results in failure, which adds to despondency. Rather than a complete, abrupt about-face from an unhealthy lifestyle, in my practice, gradual substitution of marijuana for alcohol was encouraged.

Many alcoholics use pot without consideration of it's therapeutic benefits. So, for them, the idea of increasing marijuana use while decreasing alcohol intake was not difficult. Although, with hindsight, I realize it must have been surprising to have a counselor suggest that smoking a joint instead of drinking a beer was a good idea. The biggest problem is that most alcoholics believe that marijuana is just another bad habit. Once the truth was explained to them, and if they truly wanted to stop abusive drinking, substitution of marijuana became acceptable. I was just a catalyst for their change.

By emphasizing marijuana in place of drinking at specific times, but not at all times, many of my alcoholic clients automatically increased awareness of the reasons for desiring alcoholic stupor. Pot fulfilled the "good habit as a substitution for a bad one" requirement and it helped ease the symptoms of withdrawal which are often insurmountable. To be honest, only three or four of my clients were able to stop drinking completely. They were all regular marijuana smokers before I knew them. If I had to do it over again, I would be much more direct. As it was, I only encouraged marijuana as therapy, ever so subtly.

In the framework of holistic health, alcoholism is not an incurable illness. To call it a disease is to acknowledge the extreme disequilibrium alcoholism causes for the person and the family. But in this culture, once we name something a "disease," we are expected to relinquish all control and become the obedient patient. Any personal responsibility for the disease is lifted. In the treatment of alcoholism, this disservice to the patient is magnified when the alcoholic assumes complete helplessness and hopelessness. Instead of being encouraged to change old habits through self-awareness, the medical model of conventional health care disregards the need for, and potential of, altering, at least at first, small parts of unhealthy habits and instead accepts unconsciousness as absolute and eternal. Marijuana Therapy, however, awakens us to the existence of our inner potential and allows us to sense a dimension of life that is deeper than the material.

Yoga psychology is the accumulated wisdom of thousands of years. Self-knowledge is its basic teaching. All the tools and techniques that aid in the growth of consciousness were recognized and revered long ago. Marijuana was considered a *gift of the gods* to help human life toward ever-greater understanding. Just as it worked 5000 years ago, this ancient medicine for the body, mind, and spirit is working today and is being rediscovered by health care providers and patients alike.

Alcoholism has often been called the sickness of the soul because those who succumb are usually overly sensitive to the loss of Divine purpose in today's world. In this regard, Marijuana Therapy can help the addict regain connection with Timeless Values – if only the truth be known.

Asthma

The Holistic Model of dis-ease is actually based upon ancient philosophy (rediscovered and renamed) that human life is composed of Body, Mind, and Soul. The body is only the visible representation of a whole person. The mind is the finest instrument, but the soul is the source of life. The unencumbered body and the clearest mind allow for recognition of that which abides beyond the physical and mental realities. A healthy soul is the goal of all spiritual disciplines and a requirement for the serenity sought in Holistic Health. Toward that end, breath is either a help or hindrance.

Our manner of breathing is consistent with our general level of health and well-being. It reflects the degree of harmony between the inner being and the outer personality. "The breath affects more than the body for the rhythms of the body in turn affect one's emotional and mental life. In yoga science the breath is considered to be the main link between body and mind" (Ajaya, 1983, p.193). By attaining a "pure" breath we integrate the exposed self with the secret self. Marijuana can facilitate this synthesis through its balancing effect on the Autonomic Nervous System (ANS), which regulates breathing.

Quiet, slow, sure, without ripple or pause, with depth and consistency – such a breathing pattern assures that we are centered/balanced, and at one with ourselves. In today's confounded social setting such a breath is rare. "Most people are poor breathers. Their breathing is shallow and they have a tendency to hold their breath in any situation of stress which increases tension" (Lowen,1970, p. 38). Through interest, patience, and one-pointed determination, practiced in solitude, in silent meditation, with the aid of the "sacred Bhang" the Science of Breath was formulated, in and about India over 5000 years ago by the early Hindu seekers.

Although with the stressors of modern life, breathing irregularities have escalated as evidenced by the increase of respiratory dysfunctions. The ancient traditions recognized the significance of full and unobstructed patterns of breath, whereas modern science does not. According to Dr. Andrew Weil (1990):

Breathing...is not information I got in medical school. I learned

*nothing about breathing as the bridge between mind and body,
the connection between consciousness and unconsciousness,
the movement of spirit in matter...[or that] breath is the master key
to health and wellness...A great many teachings from such
diverse traditions as yoga, martial arts, Native American religion,
natural childbirth and osteopathic medicine all point to breath as
the most important function of life.* (p. 84)

Biologically speaking, the ANS connects conscious and unconscious desires. Chronic conflict presents itself in the body as a "psychosomatic" disease which develops over time because ANS imbalance results in either *over* or *under* secretions of body chemicals – chronically.

An asthma attack is a sudden obstruction of the airway. The bronchial tubes become so severely constricted (through contraction of the muscles that surround the bronchiole) that an asthmatic patient cannot breathe! The attack is triggered (on the physical plane) by the release of histamines from specialized cells, without the corresponding appropriate release of antihistamines. Holistic practitioners perceive that the root cause of this problem is attributable to the "asthmatic personality" (and to a lesser degree, the "allergic personality type") who habitually overreacts emotionally, but without awareness, to the point that ANS functioning is chronically, dangerously destabilized. Conventional medicine, on the other hand, perceives the symptoms as being induced by substances in the air (allergens) that affect only certain people – without the reason being of concern to allopathic doctors or, as in the psychiatric explanation, caused by repressed resentment (for which amelioration of symptoms are not specifically addressed).

Once an asthma attack begins, indicating that hidden disharmony is being expressed, additional body responses kick in, which further impairs breathing. Since stale air is trapped inside the lung and the airway is constricted, the asthmatic must forcibly expel the old gas to make room for new, oxygenated air. This severe coughing (paroxysm) takes a great deal of energy and is totally exhausting, because expiration is inherently a reaction to inspiration: air that is inhaled is automatically exhaled. Forced expiration causes the diaphragm to be pushed up (more than usual) which then pulls the ribs in closer. The frantic attempt to help oneself is instinctive, yet futile; it exacerbates the problem, for the chest cavity becomes diminished in size. The area available for expansion of the lung is decreased. At the same time, with constriction of the bronchiole, the usual upward and outward expectorant movement is constrained. Mucus buildup occurs, which further hampers the breathing process. The amount of mucus increases and becomes thicker than usual because specialized mucus-producing cells within the lung are activated during the asthmatic attack.

Conventional medical treatment is progressively aggressive. Antihistamine administration at the site may serve the child. Epinephrine (adrenaline, a strong stimulant) inhalants are successful for suppressing the acute attack (as are injections for faster relief of symptoms). However, caution is recommended as anxiety and tachycardia may result from this treatment. According to Dr. Grinspoon (1971), caution has only recently been emphasized since it is now realized that aggressive conventional treatment for asthma has, in fact, been associated with many deaths.

Standard prophylactic treatment of asthma includes oral epinephrine (adrenaline), with possible use of sedatives to combat side effects (taken with caution so as not to depress respiration dangerously). Tranquilizers may also be prescribed on an "as needed" basis for the panic that accompanies the realization that one can have an attack at any moment. Cough medicines are also administered, but not too much, so as to avoid depressing the cough reflex. When all else fails, adreno-cortical steroids are employed which, after only a few months, can have devastating side effects:

> Steroids cause allergies and inflammation to disappear as if by magic. In fact, the magic is nothing other than direct suppression of immune function. I have no objection to giving these strong drugs for very severe or life-threatening problems, but even then I think they should be limited to short-term use. Steroids are terribly toxic, cause dependence, suppress rather than cure disease, and reduce the chance of healing by natural methods of treatment. Moreover, they weaken immunity. (Weil, 1990, p. 193)

And finally, after prolonged treatment with all of the above, drug tolerance/resistance sets in and oxygen-inhalants are life saving. Needless to say, each progressive step to suppress bodily symptoms causes increased undesirable and unhealthy effects.

Conventional asthma treatments are delivered to the location of each symptom, the farthest point from its cause. An apt analogy would be distributing lifejackets after a flood, rather than maintaining the damnsite to prevent a flood in the first place. Of course, once the waters break through, life jackets save lives just as inhalers and injections, etc., save lives during an asthma attack. The person can breathe again, panic diminishes, and the body slowly begins to restabilize (to an increasingly skewed familiarity). But if this keeps happening – time after time – the entire infrastructure is compromised. That is to say, like the unattended damn which gives way, the integrity of all the body systems are degraded and they collapse.

Marijuana as medicine works differently in that its performance is on the ANS, the site of the origin of the asthma attack. It not only stops an attack (at its inception) but also helps prevent further attacks by consistently balancing the two sides of the ANS (Sympathetic and Parasympathetic). Over time, it may expose the hidden psychological agendas that predispose a patient toward asthma in the first place. Marijuana affects the whole process that causes histamine overproduction at the origin of confusion, because it works on the *source* of the disturbance. The Hypothalamus portion of the brain directs the ANS and provides the perfect receptor-site, or "keyhole," for the THC molecule.

Marijuana Therapy is nonaggressive and noninvasive. It intercepts and reorders the life-threatening message *before* it is sent. It works directly at the source, and, since it is not a drug (because it has no toxicity or addictive properties, owing to its simultaneous capacity to sedate and stimulate, and is not overly concentrated by a manufacturing process), marijuana has no rebound/resistance/tolerance downside and therefore remains effective over time.

More importantly, marijuana expands lung capacity. We breathe more deeply and slowly. When taken regularly, the lungs retain that expanded capacity. Its efficacy does not diminish over the long-term, because there is no rebound, resistance, or tolerance. Marijuana affects the ANS almost immediately by causing bronchiole expansion. Histamine production is appropriately slowed or halted. Skeletal muscles in the chest are likewise relaxed through ANS mediation. The person can breathe again and peace is restored. Expectorant activation increases because marijuana improves smooth muscle motility which moves the fluids up and out of the lung – one of the main reasons cannabis-based cough medicine was so popular before synthetic medications replaced it at the pharmacy.

Using marijuana as a medical agent does not imply smoking. It can be ingested in other forms, such as the tincture of marijuana that was popular in the 19th and early 20th century for a host of health problems. Dosage can be stabilized in tinctures. The total prohibition of research has stopped its use in modern medicine. According to Dr. Grinspoon (1993), science could develop an inhalant for THC if only the ban on research were lifted.

The hidden agendas within the psyche responsible for psychosomatic disease can be exposed with regular marijuana use. Over the long term, amelioration of the symptoms of asthma through Marijuana Therapy may very well be joined to mitigation of the root cause. (Of course, we will never know whether this is an actuality, unless studies are conducted over the long term to test this hypothesis – and made public to those whose lives could be dramatically improved.) Remember: disturbances that remain hidden cannot be dealt with, but when exposed their power to disturb is seriously diminished.

I would like to say that these explanations are very simplified and have not yet been verified in "scientific" experiments; although the most progressive representatives of modern medicine admit to the efficacy of Marijuana Therapy (because the results are so overwhelmingly positive), they do not acknowledge that basic ANS balance is restored. In fact, conventional medical thinking has not addressed the issue of ANS imbalance as a cause of disease at all. Psychosomatic disease remains in the realm of "theory" from the standpoint of allopathic medicine although it is the main basis underlying Holistic Health. In the future I hope to provide more technical explanations and information about the Holistic Health Model and its interface with Marijuana Therapy as well as more detailed explanation about psychosomatic personality types and how Marijuana Therapy benefits them. I invite anyone who has had experience with marijuana and illness to send their story to Lifeservices, P.O. Box 4314, Boca Raton, FL 33429.

Chemotherapy and Nausea

In 1995 *Life Sciences* released a summary of the medical studies dealing with children with cancer who had been given marijuana to relieve the nausea and vomiting associated with chemotherapy. In total, there were 480 subjects. The results are unquestionably extremely favorable, and could (and should) easily be called "miraculous." It is well known that chemotherapy usually causes intense nausea, invariably followed by violent vomiting and, of course, complete loss of appetite. The *Life Sciences* studies reported that all 480 youngsters, ranging in age from three to thirteen, responded positively to the therapeutic administration of Delta-8-tetrahydrocannabinol: "Vomiting was completely prevented. The side effects observed were negligible."

Chemotherapy is a medical euphemism for "poisoning," the rationale of which is that cancer cells multiply exceedingly rapidly and therefore tend to metabolize the poison faster than normal cells, thus being destroyed more, and more quickly, than the integrity of the entire organism – that is, unless the poisoning happens to destroy the body or demoralize the patient past the point of affirming life. From the holistic standpoint, the rationale for poisoning the patient is completely untenable. However, conventional "wisdom" continues to employ this technique of systematically attacking the symptoms of disease rather than altering the cause or encouraging lifestyles that prevent the problem.

The substances that are used to halt or at least slow the proliferation of cancer cells (called "antineoplastic agents") are extremely toxic to the system, and understandably cause the patient to feel very sick:

> You have to understand that chemotherapy-induced nausea is not an upset tummy. It is absolutely debilitating. I wound up curled up in a ball in the fetal position, covered with my own vomit. It is such a violent action. You just keep heaving and heaving...and your system just erupts – just overwhelming physical agony.
> (Ralph Seeley, Feb. 96)

Common sense tells us that those who endure this treatment – especially children – ought to be afforded anything and everything that can alleviate their suffering. Our own Dr. Grinspoon came to the cause of Marijuana Therapy when he witnessed the miraculous effect it had on his son who underwent chemotherapy. With just a little bit of marijuana the nausea was gone, the desire to eat returned, and, naturally, "the spirit was lifted." The 1995 report from *Life Sciences* demonstrates that all children who must undergo chemotherapy may well benefit in like manner. In fact, to keep this therapy from suffering children is criminal.

The title of the article, *An Efficient New Cannabinoid Antiemetic in Pediatric Oncology,* is somewhat of a misnomer, for cannabis is certainly not new in the treatment of nausea and vomiting, since it was used for thousands of years by the ancient cultures in Egypt, Asia, and India. We are just now at the brink of major rediscovery of this natural remedy.

To understand why marijuana is perhaps the best medicine for chemotherapy-induced nausea and vomiting, we can turn again to Ralph Seeley:

> I would be getting these chemicals pumped into my veins on Friday night... Saturday and Sunday and sometimes even Monday or even Tuesday, this nausea just comes on without warning. You're just retching and you can't stop. Legal medication is in the form of pills which is very ineffective in a vomiting patient. You take one of the damn tablets and it just comes right back up.
>
> Now, you smoke a little marijuana, you get relief within 2-3 minutes...Secondly, you don't have to get that super dose. [whereas] on 5 milligrams of Marinol, it makes you very, very high and unable to concentrate and unable to do your work...[with marijuana] you feel a little bit high, the nausea recedes...there's no hangover.

From so many testimonials, regarding so many ailments, told by people from all walks of life, in all different eras and from every country in the world, we can see that Marijuana Therapy is not just an ancient remedy prescribed by what, in our arrogance, we call "primitive" cultures. In the 18th, 19th, and early 20th century, *Cannabis indica* and *Cannabis sativa* were included in the Pharmacopoeias and Materia Medicas of allopaths and homeopaths alike in all the English-speaking countries; they were also included in the herbal lore of South America, Africa and Native American cultures:

> Many people may be unaware that herbal medicine served as the primary mode of medical practice in the United States until almost 1935. This practice did change as chemical medicine burst on the scene prior to 1935...for perhaps two thousand years, all plain

physicians accepted and adhered to the...herbal...traditional systems. Yet this tremendous consensus among prominent medical authorities for two millennia is ignored. (Christi, 1988)

Nausea and lack of appetite are two of the primary uses for which cannabis was recommended in the 19th century. From the *Materia Medica* by Ruddock (1974) we learn: "*Cannabis sativa* is cause for increasing the appetite, quelling the symptoms of nausea."

As a matter of fact, the medicinal uses for which cannabis has been effective over the course of human evolution, from all I have studied, are limitless.

These age-old benefits can no longer be easily ignored since modern treatments often result in the need for increasingly larger and more lethal doses of drugs, culminating in loss of efficiency at best and horrendous, often non-reversible, problems in numerous cases. A second reason for the revival of more natural, less drastic remedies is the upsurge in information to a public eager to save the escalating cost of conventional medicine, especially with the realization that modern science often fails despite its technologies.

When it is poisoned, an organism automatically contracts. The cells are robbed of oxygen. The system becomes depressed. Even the workings of the brain are deranged. Marijuana Therapy acts to expand the entire body/mind by its autonomic investment – i.e., breathing becomes more efficient, allowing the cells to be re-oxygenated, thereby aiding in the elimination of the toxins. The dilation of blood vessels, the relaxation of the muscles, and the increased bifurcated fueling of the brain all work in symphonic harmony so that the entire system is rebalanced. The full extent of the action of marijuana on the organism is one of release of all tension – mental and physical – and easily translates into life-affirming needs, such as the desire for food.

The fact that the results of the *Life Sciences* studies with children were so favorable –"without any observable side effects" – leads us to realize that the occasional unpleasant side effects, reported in adult populations treated with Marijuana Therapy, is probably due to anxiety caused by devious brainwashing that we have been subjected to for the past half century. It is to their credit that the authors of the *Life Sciences* article realized that, without prior prejudice, medical marijuana would probably not be accompanied by any unpleasantness at all: "We chose to administer delta-8-THC to children...[it] was the general [but not documented] belief that most side effects of delta-9-THC, in particular anxiety, are more prevalent in an adult population."

As is usual in clinical treatment, before any drug is administered to human subjects, animal testing is first done. In this case, monkeys, dogs, rats, and cats were given high doses of various isomers of cannabinoids. The data indicated effective antiemetic properties as well as safety. The children were given delta-8-THC by mouth before the start of anti-cancer treatment – every six hours for 24 hours. In preliminary experiments on eight children, the clinicians stopped administering the cannabinoid after the first or second dose. "Vomiting stopped in most cases."

Therefore, in the actual test, the children were given four doses for a full 24 hours which resulted in no vomiting whatsoever. This result was in keeping with those reported in modern research articles: "Cannabinoids are currently useful therapeutically to ameliorate the nausea and vomiting of cancer chemotherapy" (Borison, 1981).

That scientific experiments showing the specific benefits of Marijuana Therapy are becoming more prevalent should give us hope to continue our struggle for its accepted medical use. However, the public access to these findings still remains difficult since they are published only in scientific journals that lay people rarely can access without the ability to understand and to interpret the medical jargon, as well as to find the appropriate medical libraries. But progress is constant and is becoming widespread as more and more of us push harder and harder to stop the censorship that exists in the mainstream media from book publishers to radio and TV talk shows, and includes the newspaper monopolies. Another ray of hope exists because, while the lay public is only beginning to suspect the miracle of this wondrous, natural, health-giving balancer of the human system, the medical world is becoming increasingly unable to ignore this reality. This is especially true among specialists, such as those in the field of cancer research and treatment.

In a random sample of over 1000 oncologists, in a survey taken to determine attitudes toward employing marijuana in treatment, revealed that more than half of those practicing physicians knew that marijuana worked in many cases where no conventional drug could. More to the point, nearly 25% of the oncologists surveyed were willing to admit that they had in the past recommended marijuana to their patients despite its illegality. These doctors for the most part represented the younger age groups, having graduated medical school in the late 60s, 70s, and 80s. "Of the respondents who expressed an opinion, a majority (54%) thought marijuana should be available by prescription," and, according to Dr. Ivan Silverberg (from the *Life Sciences* study), "there has evolved an unwritten but accepted standard of treatment within the oncologic community which readily accepts marijuana's use."

> Oncologists may prefer to prescribe smoked marijuana over oral THC for several reasons. The bio-availability of THC absorbed through the lungs has been shown to be more reliable than that of THC absorbed through the gastrointestinal tract, smoking offers patients the opportunity to self-titrate dosages to realize therapeutic levels with a minimum of side effects, and there are active agents in the crude marijuana that are absent from the pure synthetic THC. (*Life Sciences*)

This conclusion is in keeping with a very recently uncovered study done in 1978 by the New Mexican State Department of Health: *Report of the Lynn Pierson Therapeutic Research Program*. This was a controlled study with 169 human volunteers which demonstrated: (1) efficacy of marijuana to reduce the nausea and vomiting associated with chemotherapy when conventional medicines had failed; and (2) the superiority of smoked marijuana vs. the ingestion of the synthetic THC pill (Marinol) in reducing vomiting to a statistically significant degree. Prior familiarity did not lessen the effectiveness of Marijuana Therapy for nausea or vomiting, i.e., no tolerance to marijuana existed from the point of view of medical efficaciousness; and the feeling of being high was also not a factor, i.e., some patients just stopped vomiting but reported no change in consciousness.

Glaucoma

"Glaucoma is in many ways a mysterious disease process. It is more than merely the reflection of IOP or a fluid deficit or a change in the optic nervehead."
—Keith Green

In my research for this book, I was dismayed and repelled by the the vast numbers of sentient beings – cats, dogs, mice, geese, rabbits and monkeys – that were tortured and killed for the sake of human progress. By the early 70s, the medical profession already knew that smoking marijuana could be a significant remedy for glaucoma. Cannabis caused a dramatic decrease in pressure within the chambers of the eye, a pressure that, otherwise, all too often results in blindness. Many tests were launched to discover the exact mechanics of how each unique cannabinoid worked, so that their "mystery" could be understood and the essential healing substance within the marijuana plant could be synthesized and controlled. The eyes of thousands of animals were drugged and dissected in scientific laboratories and the experimental results were reported in detail in a zealous attempt to reduce the synergistic psycho-biological process of "seeing" and its interface with marijuana to the least common denominator.

Underlying these reductionistic methods is a philosophy that considers *Homo sapiens* to be superior to – and independent from – the total creation. Conventional medicine manipulates the surroundings to accommodate this illusion of separation and strives to suppress the symptoms of an unbalanced philosophy and way of life. There is little practical concern for future manifestations of a yet greater disequilibrium, except in the laboratories where animals are constantly sacrificed in the search to synthesize new drugs.

Holistic healing strives to reverse the causes of instability in the physical and emotional life, helping a patient connect with the environment, thereby harmonizing the whole person. Ironically, despite all the vivisection (or as I'd like to think, *because* of it), marijuana's beneficial effect on glaucoma has remained mysterious.

The verb "to see" describes an extremely sophisticated process by which we sense or detect the outer world through a complicated interpretation of radiant energy in the frequency of visible light. "To see" also connotes mental cognition which stems from the anatomical fact that the organ of sight is the most evolved – and the most recently evolved – outgrowth of the human brain. The optic nerve (which sees) is an "outpouching" from the forebrain and is identical in tissue composition to the brain. This sensitive and incredibly sophisticated extension of the "seat of the intellect" travels toward the exterior surface of the body to sense or "see" the outer surrounding and to relay the data back to the brain for interpretation. We should note that 40% of all sensory input to the brain comes from our eyes.

For such a complicated and fragile process as sight to succeed: the *medium* through which it operates, the *appendages* by which it is protected, and the *system* from which it is nourished and cleansed must all function in intricate interdependence. This happens within an unimaginably tiny area, made of minute capillaries of nourishment and microscopic cavernous channels of drainage which are all in profound and constant communication with each other, always invested with direction from the brain's interpretation of what is needed at any given moment.

Aqueous Humor, The Medium of Nourishment

The eyeball is filled with a clear, watery fluid called the *Aqueous Humor* and separated into two main compartments, the *Anterior Chamber,* a small elliptical slit between the iris and the cornea, and the *Posterior Chamber,* which makes up the remaining portion. The Aqueous fluid, which is electromagnetically charged to transmit light, is in constant flux, being produced in the Posterior Chamber in the "ciliary process," flowing into the Anterior Chamber and then draining into the "trabecular meshwork" (channels of drainage). Constancy of pressure, as well as the appropriate metabolic composition for nourishment and cleansing of surrounding tissues, is maintained by a dynamic tension in the Aqueous Humor which serves also as a protective envelope for the fragile optic nervehead. The integrity of the shape of the eyeball is further sustained by the Aqueous.

In glaucoma, the eyeball (in all its functions) degenerates when the intraocular pressure (IOP) rises beyond the limits of tolerance for the optic nerve, causing irreversible damage and blindness. Ultimately, glaucoma is a failure of the brain's attempt to sense the outer world and make sense of it.

In the philosophy of holistic healing, all disease is rooted in functional cause. We may speculate that the brain, in its interpretation of what it sees, is "distressed," and that stress is reflected in the IOP rise or tension within the eyeball. This fits well with another speculation that the optic nervehead itself may be undernourished, thereby causing the problem.

The Glaucomatous Process

An increase in Intraocular Pressure (IOP) beyond safe limits, sometimes suddenly, but usually gradually, with progressive vision failure, defines glaucoma. The rise in intraocular tension is related to an *imbalance* between the *production of Aqueous* and its *drainage* through normal exit channels. Production of Humor is continuous and is refurbished completely every one to two hours. Drainage is likewise continuous and in the healthy eye; the drainage out should equal the flow in. The medical consensus is that obstruction exists inside and at the beginning of the drainage channels. Whether the imbalance is explained as too much fluid, or too little drainage, the end result is irreversible blindness unless remedied.

The Marijuana Remedy

Within about one hour after smoking marijuana, and for the four to five hours following, the IOP within the eyeball is dramatically reduced to safe limits even in the extremely high pressure associated with the latter stages of glaucoma. The drainage routes dilate and reduced tension is echoed in the ciliary body which results in less call for aqueous formation. By Parasympathetic innervation, the outflow channels are relaxed and dilated. "There is an increased …permeability," according to Dr. Keith Green (1976), glaucoma's foremost research scientist. And by Parasympathetic action, the inflow channels are constricted: "Vasoconstriction of the afferent feeder vessels of the ciliary body causes a pressure fall in the capillaries." Dr. Green continues:

"This effect occurs concurrently and paradoxically by a mechanism which is not yet understood."

Because marijuana "sedates and stimulates" (as it was described over 100 years ago in the Indian Hemp Drugs Commission Report), it has a balancing effect on the Automatic Nervous System (ANS) that is unique and actually unstudied in Western medicine. This "balancing" effect has caused major confusion regarding how marijuana benefits so many stress-related diseases, in general, and glaucoma, in particular. Confusion has resulted in untold experiments aimed at understanding the *one* way that Marijuana Therapy alleviates the IOP increases associated with glaucoma.

But Marijuana Therapy works in *two* ways – on both sides of the ANS – as no other known substance does (i.e. "paradoxically!"). Until this is "seen" in the cognitive sense (which is very difficult in the current medical framework of Either/Or drugs, instead of Both/And), and its importance understood, the working of Marijuana Therapy will remain an enigma.

First, the "miosis" (pupil constriction) effect of marijuana through the Parasympathetic side of the ANS causes less straining "to see," signifying a relaxed organ of sight compared to "End Stage Glaucoma" (when no hope is left) the pupil is as dilated as possible in a futile attempt to impact a degenerated optic nerve.

Second, the drainage of aqueous is integrated into the sinus drainage areas where the mucus is thinner and more motile with marijuana (note the article on Asthma, p. 89). Studies also show an increase of protein content of the humor with marijuana use, suggesting less need for more fluid as well as an increase of sodium transport because of increased tissue permeability.

Actually, glaucoma is a problem of increased blood pressure within the eye. Marijuana has been shown to lower blood pressure within the whole body, including the eye. We should again be reminded:

> *As it is not proper to try to cure the eyes without the head, nor the head without the body, so neither is it proper to cure the body without the soul, and this is the reason why so many diseases escape physicians who are ignorant of the whole.* —Plato

Experiments with Marijuana

At first I welcomed the June 21, 1995 JAMA, article that finally recognized and encouraged further testing of marijuana because of its "medical promise," until I realized those studies would entail research through vivisection of countless animals. In a typical laboratory experiment, the autonomic nerves that travel to the eye were severed, "ganglionectomized," in hundreds of animals. THC, extracted from the natural marijuana plant, was shown to lower the pressure in their eyeballs, even though the animals were alive and awake with their heads clamped in a vise! Of course, the THC didn't work nearly as well as before the maiming, when the local auto-nomic nerves were in place, but the decrease in IOP was still significant. The results of the study were also confusing since it was unclear how THC injected into the body affected the IOP when the *local* autonomic optic nerves were cut off. The researchers also discovered that nothing happened when THC was injected directly into the brain, suggesting no interface between marijuana and the Central Nervous System (CNS), or even the ANS, which is impos-sible.

It is my hypothesis that the whole body/mind effects of Marijuana Therapy provides more oxygenated blood to the brain (and there-fore to the optic nerve), not by CNS mediation, but by ANS balancing through the systemic Hypothalamic molecular interface with THC (and not the *local* autonomic nerve sites). Therefore we see better, and think better because we are less threatened and therefore less in the constricted mode. The optic nerve in medical studies is understood as in need of nourishment, cleansing, and protection, but the psychological component of "seeing" and its connection to glaucoma is thus far unrecognized and unstudied.

"The notion that ocular damage," Dr. Green points out, "depends on an imbalance of intraocular pressure and blood supply to the optic nerve...shifts the emphasis from IOP to the anatomic and physiologic state of the optic nerve."

Unfortunately, standard scientific experiments not only dissect helpless animals, but also dissect and extract individual compounds from the marijuana plant that "show promise" as potential synthetic pharmaceuticals, notably: cannabinoid, cannabidiol, cannabinoic acid, cannabigerol, cannabicicyclol, and the isomers of THC – Delta 1, 8 & 9. The entire point of the wholesome delivery of nature's herbal tonic is therefore circumvented, and the results of each specific extract have either less beneficial effect than the intact plant or no beneficial effect at all.

According to Dr. Green et al. (1976), "Awareness that marijuana lowered IOP has spurned a great effort to identify the mechanism by which this effect occurs, and [provide a] delivery system to the eye which can lower IOP without the well-known psychotropic side effects."

The Holistic Understanding

Mind (as the finest instrument of human processing) operates through the mechanical processes of the brain and "goes out" to experience, see, and interpret the surroundings. The natural propensity and main function of the brain is to serve as a vehicle by which the individual consciousness can realize (by its relationship with the world) itself. In this understanding, the optic nerve is the organ whereby nearly half of all data is detected to be deciphered and interpreted by the mind through the brain. The task of protection, nourishment, and cleansing are relegated to the automatic processes of balance, allowing for the higher centers to focus on more complex decisions.

In the ancient science of the Medicine of India (Ayurveda) organs degenerate because of overuse, underuse, or misuse. To simplify: in the glaucomatous process what is seen is interpreted disfavorably by the brain, the ANS responds accordingly, creating tension in the face of a perceived threat. If this reaction is long-standing, without relief, the organ degenerates. Chronic imbalance is chronic tension. There is no doubt in my mind that glaucoma is a psychosomatic disorder. However, it is also obvious to me that some form of outward intervention is needed other than knowing one ought to relax. So far, only Marijuana Therapy serves all the parameters of subtlety needed for relief of the complicated symptoms of glaucoma to alter or reveal the root cause of the tension. One researcher (Flom, 1975) intuited this connection between marijuana and glaucoma: "Analysis suggests an indirect effect ... associated with relaxation."

Discussion

Just because marijuana can work so effectively is no reason for using it, if pharmaceutical medicines were as good or better. The original reason marijuana lost favor was because its results were considered too variable, and our modern medical science demanded predictability.

> Pharmaceutical treatments are predictable all right: after many years of research, NONE of them work as safely or as effectively as Marijuana Therapy, nor are they as easy to self-medicate in appropriate dosage. (Grinspoon, 1995)

Furthermore, in glaucoma research, Dr. Green (1976) reports that for marijuana use: "studies indicate that the IOP fall is as good or better than most agents."

The fact that no control is necessary (because there is no danger of an overdose) and that individual patient control of dosage is better than the objective determination of a physician, represents the problem that marijuana poses to the authority of the doctor, in contrast to the autonomy and sense of self-determination it affords the patient.

Marijuana is *constant* in its complete harmlessness and its absolute healthfulness. It has no deleterious side effects that researches can identify except the psychological component of feeling "high," which is mistakenly deemed a negative.

In some studies of marijuana, there was a lowering of blood pressure in the whole body upon first-time use that was uncomfortable, called "postural hypotension," where the patient needed to lie down for a few minutes to alleviate the feeling of faintness. Perhaps this extreme hypotension (which was momentary and only occurred upon the first-time experience) was caused by the fear that accompanies "seeing" things as they really are and perhaps being uncomfortable with the loss of defense mechanisms.

Other adverse effects noted are anxiety (which, of course, is related to the fear of psychological nakedness), feeling hungry and thirsty (the munchies), and experiencing an increased heart rate. However, one study showed that a single marijuana cigarette worked effectively, even when more had previously been used. This supports the "less is more" theory, a brilliant technical explanation given by John Gettman (1995), *Marijuana & the Brain, Part II: The*

Tolerance Factor.

On the other hand, the approved treatments for glaucoma are all dangerous to overall health, are fraught with horrendous side effects, and must be monitored continuously for life-threatening dangers. They are, however, completely controllable by the doctor, and precise doses of drugs are predictably available by prescription from the pharmaceutical giants at great cost to the patient.

The side effects of the conventional medicines, in contrast to the benign or beneficial aspects of marijuana, are numerous. Furthermore, as the treatment proceeds over time, synthetic medicines must be constantly altered. In fact, the longer one takes these "medicines," the more necessary it becomes to either increase dosage or switch to ever more dangerous drugs.

Some of the most noteworthy and common side effects of approved medical treatment for glaucoma include: headaches, drug allergy, metabolic acidosis, rashes, cataracts, hypotension, blood dyscrasia, kidney stones, and ulcers. When the synthetic pharmaceutical medicines fail – as they all do over time, owing to their one-sidedness which assures tolerance – more aggressive medicines are employed whose side effects include hallucinations, anxiety, mania, bone marrow depletion, retinal detachment, cardiovascular bradycardia, and, finally, death from respiratory failure.

When all else fails and blindness is imminent, surgical opening of the outflow channels is attempted. The success rate is: three out of 11 surgical patients wake up blind. In two to three weeks, another two or three patients will become blind. If they have open-angle glaucoma, a progressively deleterious disease, chances are about 50/50 that patients will go blind over time.

With Marijuana Therapy, however, a successful cure is almost always guaranteed.

Multiple Sclerosis

We tend to believe that the ban on testing marijuana has resulted in a lack of documentation of its effects. But such is not the case. In the scientific literature, there exist thousands of studies that have investigated distinct elements of cannabis in relationship to human physiology. These "cannabinoids" have been analyzed extensively in order to learn the secret mechanism of how they affect (the artificially separated components of) our constitutions. Each part of the puzzle of human reactivity to different cannabis compounds stands alone and, so far, there is no acknowledgment of what these isolated discoveries suggest for the case of Marijuana Therapy.

In modern science, the only acceptable method for testing a drug is the "double-blind" investigation which assures objective determination of how a substance impacts on an organism at that time and place. Only the pharmaceutical companies are allowed to perform double-blind studies with marijuana because it is classified as a Schedule I Drug (the most dangerous type, without recognized medical value). The sinister agreement with the government (1976) was that only the pharmaceutical industry would be allowed to test marijuana for a 10-year period, during which time a synthetic would be developed that would fulfill the recognized medical promise of cannabis without the psychoactive properties. Needless to say, this effort has not succeeded; neither has the ban been lifted to allow for the double-blind testing that science accepts as valid as was promised.

In direct contrast to *objective* science, the ancient disciplines not only made note of the obvious effects of a remedy, but also amassed detailed descriptions of each patient's *subjective* experience. Since conscious regulation of one's own state of health was a sacred responsibility, primary respect was given to experiential assessment. Holistic medicine is the modern equivalent of this philosophy which encourages awareness of one's own body/mind in relationship to its surroundings.

Since the double-blind study is the only acceptable form of testing a medicine's efficiency, the medical community has itself become blind to the validity of individual testimony, even when vast numbers of individuals report similar benefits. Unconscious resistance to reason is the leading cause of Marijuana research and Therapy prohibition.

In hearings before the State of California to determine whether or not Marijuana Therapy ameliorated the symptoms of MS, the patients were sworn to tell the truth, and really had no reason whatsoever to lie, yet their "anecdotal" testimony was disregarded by the conventional health care professionals as being unscientific and therefore without value.

> Valerie Leith Cover: "Prior to smoking, I was throwing up and suffering from spasms. However, within five minutes of smoking marijuana, I stopped vomiting, no longer felt nauseous, and noticed my intense spasms were significantly reduced. The sense of "shakiness" which I constantly felt deep inside me seemed to diminish. At one point, without thinking, I stood up unaided!" (May 8, 1987)

Having been on a very high regimen of ACTH (which triggers the body to release mega-doses of its own steroids), and owing to severe and dangerous side-effects, Mr. Paufler, another MS patient, decided – *for the third time* – to stop using this medication.

> Gary Paufler: "The ACTH was making me worse and the side-effects were overwhelming me. I was bedridden. If it was a choice between this treatment, I would rather have MS. I was placed on *prednisone* (a steroid) in its place. Medical records indicate I died that day...there was a nearly total absence of potassium in my body (from taking prescribed drugs). I stopped all steroid drugs but continued using valium.
>
> "I began smoking marijuana...to get high. One evening some old friends came to visit, and we smoked several joints. When my friends got up to say good-bye, I stood up. Everybody stared. I was stunned. (Then) I walked. The longer I smoked marijuana, the better I got. My eyesight returned. I began walking, my spasms were nonexistent." (May 11, 1987)

There are many more affidavits of patients who testified at those hearings, all equally dramatic, pointing to the untold benefits of Marijuana Therapy. The reactions of two medical doctors are given:

> Dr. Kenneth P. Johnson: "The information regarding the use of marijuana...is purely anecdotal...There is no medical documentation...it is difficult to determine exactly what (the patient) claims marijuana did for him, especially in his claim that it improved his 'sense of well-being'...It is virtually impossible for any drug to cause the miraculous and immediate improvements claimed by the affiant...Each of these lay persons decided for

themselves what quantity (of marijuana) was sufficient...I must conclude that marijuana should remain in Schedule I (because) I cannot conclude that marijuana is effective in treating MS."
Dr. Donald H. Silverberg: "I have reviewed the affidavits...None are supported by scientific or medical findings... their claimed results... are useless... Further, the negative effects of using marijuana...make it unacceptable for treating MS. Second... I know of no drug...used in smokable form. Also... the use of (marijuana) especially for long term treatment would be worse than the original disease itself." (July 13, 1987)

Since MS is a disease that is treated mainly for its symptoms, the doctors have tried just about anything imaginable that might help this energetic failing – from electrical current, to diet, to vitamin therapy – in hope of spurring repair of damaged nerve fibers, they have used all range of depressants to dampen the spasticity associated with MS, and, most recently, the employment of immune suppressants to slow, or try to eliminate yet further deterioration to the nerve bundles.

The majority of conventional medicines are so concentrated as to affect the organism immediately and aggressively in hope of suppressing the symptoms of discomfort. Pharmaceutical treatment is employed nearly across the board, even though every study readily acknowledges that the intricate physical-chemical mechanisms that these concentrated drugs trigger within the patient is not understood: "studies of short term therapy with brief periods of follow-up consistently demonstrate that corticosteroids, particularly in large doses, can alter almost any aspect of the immune system. There are no studies yet on long term hazards."

The short term dangers of the corticosteroids that are known include: malignancy, irreversible reductions in immune response balance, hypertension, diabetes, anemia, renal insufficiency, venous thrombosis, herpes zoster infection, urosepsis, flu, depression, rash, blood toxicity, loss of strength, hallucination, tremor, ulcers, meningitis, hypotension, ataxia, drowsiness, heart disturbance, bone marrow suppression, seizures.

The approximate cost of *Betaseron,* the newest of these aggressive medications given to MS patients, is $10,000 per year. The total profit to its pharmaceutical manufacturer would be $645 million per year, if we assume use by 150,000 of the 250,000 MS patients in the U.S.

On the other side, far from the crowd of commercialized concentrations, is cannabis. This plant of exquisite beauty and incredible strength, of ubiquitous climatological adaptation, and of primordial connection on a cellular level with life on this planet, has been the subject of great interest and intensive study over the past several decades. Its most well-known physical effects seem especially tailored to the needs of MS patients. Sometimes, nearly miraculous abatement of the *weakness, spasticity,* and *mental depression* associated with Multiple Sclerosis has been demonstrated and is documented in the scientific literature. Buried in the research of the past 30 years are 2018 experiments with marijuana and/or its various compounds that demonstrate the scientific reasons as to HOW marijuana works to restore balance and integrate coordination in patients who are in dire need of medical help and mental hope.

The THC molecule has a unique receptor at the site of the Autonomic Nervous System which directs our involuntary body/mind reactions. Immediately upon smoking marijuana, we breathe more fully and our breath is more fully oxygenated. The severe *weakness* associated with MS is just as immediately lessened. More oxygen is delivered to the entire body – including to the atrophied or oxygen deprived muscles – which in turn feel stronger (because they are). The brain is likewise delivered more oxygen and, since THC provides a bilateral, balanced delivery to this bifurcated organ, this helps lessen symptoms of *spasticy* and *vertigo.*

In 1992, a study was reported in the Medical Journal of Australia that found: "in experienced marijuana smokers, marijuana smoking was accompanied by a significant bilateral increase in cerebral blood flow," and further on, "Marijuana is known to increase sensory awareness which may account for the increase in blood flow after marijuana use" (Caswell, 1992).

Of course, this logic is not in order. We know that enhancement of sensory awareness is a result, not a cause, of the increased blood flow to the brain. Nevertheless, this study was done according to double-blind rules and therefore proved by deduction what we already knew. More to the point, specifically in reference to MS, which has as one of its direct problems a loss of circulation in the brain capillaries, we now have proof that marijuana reverses this symptom.

According to Russel, "Tough physical training to improve the circulation in the capillaries of the CNS" is helpful for the MS patient. But without any tough physical training, a ludicrous notion for an incapacitated victim of MS, who may not be able to walk, talk, or even see, Marijuana Therapy unquestionably accomplishes this needed increase in capillary circulation.

Loss of coordination *(ataxia)* is a very common occurrence in MS; it is one of the main debilitations reported to be dramatically improved with Marijuana Therapy. In 1989, a study was done by the Federal Republic of Germany which showed that smoking marijuana:

> ... may have powerful beneficial effects on both spasticity and ataxia: the anti-spastic actions of marijuana in both clinical rating and electrophysiological testing are similar to those seen in patients after clonidine, diazepam...The important difference is that marijuana apparently also has anti-ataxic actions not described to any anti-spastic drug.

The drugs that are usually administered for MS almost invariably help one symptom while aggravating another. The drugs that decrease spasticity are depressants which, as a side effect, further the symptoms of weakness and loss of coordination. And they also have the dangerous side effects (already listed) common to one-sided drugs. Spasticity is an excessive activity of motor neurons and an associated lack of reciprocal innervation. Scientific studies discovered one of the secrets of Marijuana Therapy when they found that both THC and CBD (another cannabis compound) caused

> ...an increased firing threshold in individual neurons. Maybe cannabinoids modulate the intra-cellular metabolism and regulate the activity of multiple cellular processes.

Actually, because of the way THC affects the entire physiology (slightly increased heart rate and increased capacity of the lungs), the damaged, oxygen deprived nerves are reinvigorated or upgraded in their capacity – if not to normal, then at least to "better-than-before" capabilities. The muscle spasticity is generally relieved, owing to the relaxation of the entire musculature.

People with MS often lose sensation in their extremities. When the nerves are more fully fueled, as happens with Marijuana Therapy, this discomfort diminishes. Laboratory testing of THC demonstrated increased sensory awareness which validates what marijuana smokers have always known.

THC, however, is also defined and maligned as "psychoactive," which simply means (in functional terminology) that a person's outlook becomes fuller, broader, and more energized. We know that marijuana balances our involuntary physiology. This includes the mental depression that results from a downtrodden and narrow perspective of one's own personal situation. The "Lifting of the Spirit" that accompanies Marijuana Therapy is in perfect keeping with its scientific laboratory findings, on a cellular level – of more sensations – including clearer insight of one's predicament.

The diagnosis of MS follows a series of complicated tests which show damage to the insulation surrounding nerve fibers in the brain and in the spinal cord. Conventional treatment attempts to halt further damage by administering aggressive medications (corticosteroids) that suppress the over-active immune system which has gone askew and is thereby causing, or at least allowing, the damage. Conventional medicine is actually trying to rebalance or "modulate" this over-excited immune system.

Of course, working unilaterally and aggressively on one side of any bifurcated organic system will result in an equal rebound action, which is the reason immuno-suppressants are so dangerous. No synthetic drug has yet been manufactured that has "immune modulating" effects; instead, drugs act in an either exciting or depressing fashion. The miracle of THC in its effect on the immune system, however, has now been found to be "immuno-modulating" (Kusher, 1994). This is a significant discovery and one which suggests that marijuana is not indicated just for the symptoms of MS, but may actually help to halt its usual progression.

But marijuana imparts so much more than the effects of the well-known THC molecule. It is comprised of hundreds of unique cannabinoids which scientists have shown match or "fit" receptors in our DNA. For example, there is a receptor for CX5 (another cannabinoid) which suggests an ancient connection, a "highly conserved throughout human evolution" profile. In other words, CX5 *was an evolving companion to* human evolution.

According to the results from a study in Great Britain, "CX5 suggests a possible role in inflammatory and immune responses (because) its human receptor is on a macrophagic cell," which cells are thought to play an "immuno-modulating role." This is extremely significant in our understanding of Marijuana Therapy and its interface with MS. Tests indicate that macrophagic cells do not function properly at the site of the nerve damage in MS.

The anti-inflammatory, immunomodulating sophistication of just one cannabinoid (among hundreds) as demonstrated by the scientific community's own tests is available for all to see in university libraries in every city in the country. The increased blood flow in the brain with its resultant increase in sensitivity, coordination, sense of balance, and overall strengthening, is well documented in pharmaceutical studies. There is no scientific basis for accusing patients of not knowing what they mean when they detect a "sense of well-being."

All these chemical dissections of marijuana in the laboratory point to balancing and modulating benefits. But as we travel through these reductionistic experiments, the importance of the intact plant's interdependent molecular effects must never be forgotten. The beneficial indications of each isolated compound of cannabis are just modest whispers of what the whole and holy ancient sativa promises. But right now, the sad fact remains that seriously sick people are being denied the best medicine available, because too many doctors believe suffering from MS (or any disease) is preferable to using the herbal medicine that provides relief.

According to Dr. Grinspoon, *Marihuana: The Forbidden Medicine*, patients report that they find smoked herbal cannabis better at controlling their symptoms than synthetic derivatives, and "cannabis may even retard the progression of the disease". This is an absolutely astounding observation, and one that deserves serious and immediate study! Dr. Robert Pertwee (Dept. of Biomedical Science, Aberdeen University) wants to carry out a proper clinical trial of smoked cannabis for MS. Unfortunately, especially for MS victims, he still needs proper funding and a source for legal cannabis.

Questions/Answers/Commentary

In the course of distributing preliminary copies of this book to various reviewers, Jon Hanna (Soma Graphics, Box 19820, Sacramento, CA 95819-0820) posed a few questions that deserve in-depth answers. Jon Hanna has recently begun to review and publicize all the serious literature available on psychedelics.

Jon Hanna: "Wouldn't it be hard for a regular user of marijuana who was used to its balancing effect on the ANS to go back to the "stressful" ups and downs of a normally functioning body? Couldn't there be withdrawal symptoms associated with this? I know that my brother-in-law (a habitual, chronic marijuana smoker) who is normally an extremely easy going guy turns very cranky when he is out of pot for a few days. In an interview in "FreakBeat", No. 8, Terrence McKenna (a habitual pot smoker) relates what happened when he quit smoking pot: "... so then I did quit for two months, and what I did notice was a tremendous narrowing of my consciousness." Can a person be addicted to "higher consciousness?"

Answer: Stressful ups and downs are difficult for everyone. Stress is the reason for the unhealthy yet acceptable habits of smoking tobacco, using sugar, drinking alcohol, watching TV. If a person has found a healthy way of warding off stress, and the healthy way is then no longer available to him/her, such as jogging each day, meditating regularly, eating healthful foods, or using marijuana on a daily basis, there is no doubt that the person will feel unbalanced, cranky and normally stressed.

The issue of consciousness must be seen from a slightly different perspective. Addiction is a reaction to imbalance, which leads to none other than continued and more skewed imbalance. Consciousness is born of balance, and once the organism is out of sync, by definition, higher consciousness disappears. In order for someone who usually maintains balance through marijuana (and enjoys the attendant higher awareness born of that balance) to continue in a higher state of consciousness without marijuana, another stabilizer would be needed. Balance restored through work on oneself, such as meditation, prayer, yoga, breathing exercises, cognitive conversion, results in a raised consciousness. The practice of marijuana is not different than any other. As a student of yoga, who must constantly do his/her discipline, so must the Christian priest or nun practice prayer and partake of the sacraments as a constant lifelong discipline. In all spiritual endeavors, it is hoped that regular and continuous practice will so habituate the aspirant in warding off programs of self serving desires, that he/she will be graced with a permanent equanimity. Any transgression from the ideal is but a signpost that the practitioner must keep on working.

Jon Hanna also questioned my assessment that the "short term memory loss" associated with marijuana is a "marijuana myth." I hope I can clear up this confusion.

If you're riding in a car at 60 miles an hour, looking out the window at the scenery of mountains and trees, the attention you can pay to any one tree is very superficial. The perception you are having is through a very large "window of consciousness" (Fishkin & Jones) with a tremendous amount of stimulation being admitted, whose rate of movement is quite fast (Sympathetic Mode - Stimulation). When the car is nearly at a standstill, only one tree may be in what has now become a much smaller "window of consciousness." It will appear in greater depth because you will be taking in details not before available to your quickly moving, although larger window (Parasympathetic Mode - Relaxation).

Marijuana BOTH enlarges the window by giving a perspective that can sometimes be termed "global" AND slows down the rate of "attentional shift" (Fishkin and Jones, 1978) to a concentrated mode of intensity, sometimes to where it appears as though "time stands still." We can also understand this experience, psychologically, as the state where there is no ego or awareness of separate orchestration between oneself and the universe. It can be a magnetic experience because of its intensity.

When we deepen our intensity of attention (because we've slowed down and have time and energy to use for intensification of awareness) and also widen our window of consciousness, according to this model, a "receptive mode" (neither active or passive) is entered. In yogic science, we are said to become more "aware" and "one-pointed" in our depth of understanding the underlying reality. Life, in general feels less random, has meaning, and is interesting. These features define an *altered state of consciousness* only because it is unusual to our usual way of being (Tart, 1975). In this understanding of altered states of consciousness, less interest is paid to the common trivia of mundane existence. If we become accustomed to this sharpness of perception, as with regular marijuana use or various techniques to increase our mindfulness or consciousness, the altered state nomenclature is no longer as valid nor is the intensification of awareness as magnetic. That is why – when we overuse marijuana – we tend to feel as though we no longer "get high." Getting high assumes raising up from a lower, less full experience, and the act of raising up itself represents the altering which is sought as an event that gives a shock and thereby helps us to notice the underlying reality – which is a natural, innate, although suppressed, human need, neither recognized nor fulfilled, for the most part, in or by modern society. Instead daily life is not really all that momentous because we don't take time, have time, or even know that we need time. The overly active mode of taking in all manner of information at a very fast pace is the short-term memory "SKILL" necessarily encouraged in modern life. It is neither healthy nor natural for our organism, but it is the way to function most successfully on the treadmill of contemporary life. It is the skewed-toward-Sympathetic overload, about which this entire book was written.

When one is paying very close attention to the meaning/beauty/ function of some things, less energy or interest is available to other things, especially things without such import, which is what often happens in the marijuana experience during times where we just don't pay close attention to, for example, a conversation. This is the short-term memory disassocciation from the activity around us that can happen with marijuana. But to call it a "loss" is inappropriate because:

1. When one learns anything or notices anything while having the marijuana experience, the memory of it, as well as the present experience, is greater/keener and fuller and also easier to retrieve and less lost over time. According to Fishkin and Jones, "should memory be sampled under the influence of marijuana, it could be done with greater intensity and with a greater flow of deeper-lying or unusual associations being brought into consciousness."

2. "Loss" implies having the information as a permanent registration in the mind – which doesn't happen with marijuana "disas-

sociation". Instead there is no registration of the event to the memory bank. The deposit is never made. Only when a deposit in the bank is made will the memory of it be clearer and easier to retrieve if made while experiencing marijuana.

3. "Short-term memory loss" smacks of a senility not at all like the marijuana experience. Senility/Alzheimer Disease becomes increasingly worse over time because the window of consciousness is foggy, stuck at one point of reference, and the link between it (the window) and the long term memory storage area shorts out or becomes clogged to access – all of which can be translated into the hardening of the arteries of the brain found in autopsy reports of Alzheimer patients, even in young victims. This memory loss includes not knowing one's relatives, how to dress, or what is socially acceptable. The person actually "forgets" or loses something he/she had at a previous time.

With marijuana, the present perception and the long-term memory bank are more in communication NOT less. First, because of the greater blood flow to all areas and nerves of the brain, and second because non-verbal comprehension increases (Fishkin and Jones) which allows for the experience to be fuller or more. The meaning is clearer. "Nonverbal" corresponds to the intensification of flash understandings or intuitions. Interest in the now naturally leads away from inconsequential events and therefore can rightly be termed as a "loss of interest" of any particular occurrence. Important issues are not disregarded because marijuana affects the person in a way than enhances awareness of important issues as well as increasing the desire to be more conscientious in issues of import.

4. The "loss of interest" to certain enculturated activities (which may create lapses in attention to mundane things), while disturbing to the onlooker, is overcome simply by intentional refocusing on the subject by the person in an altered state or higher consciousness.

> A common experience for marijuana users (is) to say they can come down at will, that if they find themselves in a situation they feel unable to cope with adequately while in the altered state of consciousness of marijuana...(they) can deliberately suppress...effects. (Sugarman and Tarter, 1978)

The "loss" of interest, not of memory, can immediately evaporate during an emergency completely unlike any brain dysfunction such as Alzheimer. Remember: *the balance of marijuana is quite natural to the healthy organism.* When an emergency presents, the Sympathetic mode is immediate. From balance, the appropriate response is easily accomplished. We can liken the "disassociation" from immediate trivia that occurs with the marijuana experience as something akin to *the absent-minded-professor syndrome,* without suggesting that all marijuana experience is Einstein-like. Thousands of years ago, the Chinese prescribed cannabis to increase and maintain one's memory; so they knew then what we are just beginning to understand.

5. and, probably most important to the scientific criticism, this effect of "disassociation of interest" is immediately reversible upon discontinuance of the marijuana experience. We can also note that, as the marijuana experience or high state becomes more familiar, less disassociation will occur since the novelty of that experience is no longer quite as magnetic.

6. Finally, fear of this "loss of interest" to cultural values of extreme competitiveness scares the mainstream. This is because of a total lack of comprehension of the naturalness of being "high" and its healthfulness for our entire population and future on the planet

---

UPDATE

(8/21/97, *Nature*) Dr. Daniele Piomelli discovered a natural brain substance that seems to mimic cannabis. 2-AG (sn-2 arachidonylglycerol) is being described as a "modulator in memory formation,". The electrical sensitivity (of brain cells) changes over time (days/weeks) as any one stimulus is chosen to be remembered. 2-AG is a discriminator in what it lets the cells prepare to remember.

The discovery of 2-AG is very new. It will surely be tested in great detail as science attempts to understand the "how" of human functions. The philosophers' understanding as to the "why" consequently becomes validated: we surely can't remember every stimulus. What lets us forget what isn't even important to try to remember seems to be 2-AG. It (apparently) deactivates the exact same process in our brain cells as cannabis. To remember the important items - less important events need not even be given any mind - "pay it no mind."

Chapter 6 • The Prohibition Problem
Confessions of a Drug Counselor

As a drug counselor within a county agency, I was constantly exposed to mainstream health-care jargon. "Self-Medicating" was the derogatory label reserved for our clients' behavior, almost all of whom were attending Drug Counselling against their will as an alternative to prison. I was an imposter amidst the social work mentality that prevails within the hallowed walls of the Mental Health Community.

Friday was "case conference" day during which all the employees would gather together to ridicule a few previously-designated clients. We would sit in a circle with our coffee, cigarettes, and candy, and discuss with smug superiority the foolhardiness of all the "self-medicators." The staff was composed of our boss, who was unabashedly addicted by legal prescription to valium; two "recovering" (sometimes) alcoholics; two incredibly obese social workers; a few young interns; and me. As an imposter in psychologist costume, whose heart was with all those people who were self-medicating their dis-ease, it was infuriating to maintain my disguise. I ascribe to the unpopular, although well-recognized, thought in Humanistic Psychology that therapy walks a fragile line between mending the non-integrated personality and manipulating it to fit within the social norm. The message in today's society is to denigrate the notion of higher consciousness, despite the fact that all in-depth psychological studies recognize the value inherent in such an essential experience. Reminding my co-workers of this danger all too often set me apart from the agency's stated purpose – which was none other than to monitor and control the use of all illegal drugs by the client – and failing at that – to send the adjudicated customer directly to jail.

For the most part, the agency's clientele was under 30, and the crime was getting caught either using or selling herb. There were, of course, some who used hard drugs, whose lives were in constant upheaval. These cases were difficult. After a few years I realized there was a spiritual void which drove such destructive behavior. Only a super effort, born of undistracted interest and compassion, could touch these hard-core addicts. My own suggestion – to substitute herb for heroin had to be couched in careful phrases lest the establishment would get wind of my true identity.

Holistic health counseling shares the philosophy of Systems Theory except that the system is perceived as far broader than the term usually denotes, taking into account not only behavior, motivation, and interaction with and from the outside world, but also dealing with the subjective, universal, and deep needs of human beings, which are always of a spiritual nature, however costumed, and including the influence that the counselor not only exerts on the client but also how the client-counselor experience impacts and enriches the world of both.

In the separatist world of professional psychology, the notion of becoming friends with one's clients is taboo for it blurs the lines between the authoritarian position and the subservient state of the un-empowered. When I worked within the boundaries of the County Agency, this rule of segregation was difficult to abide by. Needless to say, I followed no such rigid formula in my own practice. "Counselor" is a "user-friendly" term to replace the arrogant, dated, nomenclature of "therapist." Holistic Health, with its main focus on self-responsibility, goes one step further to a teacher/student model. I considered myself a teacher who imparted knowledge and encouragement, and many of my former students became my friends. Holistic counseling also recognizes that what is the best direction for the three dimensions of human life (body/mind/soul) may not be the most socially acceptable. In the case of two alcoholic outcasts, this was definitely true. To overcome the numbness of alcohol, I suggested that some clients increase their regular marijuana ingestion. Additional use of marijuana proved to be very good medicine as well as a wonderful aid to concentrating the mind for study. My students, who had been inebriated for so long, began to awaken from their stupor.

If alcoholics can learn to take in progressively more pot and less booze, at some point the individual consciousness reasserts itself and the mechanical drive to be drunk, along with all its pitfalls, becomes a conscious, controllable desire instead of a self-propelling reaction.

The therapeutic 50-minute hour was often uplifing, despite the troubled life situations of my subjects. It was refreshing to share the mental set of these non-programmed "criminals" who had dared to self-medicate themselves and their friends, and who were consequently policed by the state. Urine testing was mandatory, and supposed to be a surprise. It's interesting to note that urinalysis is only truly effective in detecting psychedelic plants, since all the hard (manufactured) drugs (including alcohol) are metabolized in a few days. The client need only stop "using" 48 hours before the counseling session, then his/her test will show "clean." It's also noteworthy that a doctor's prescription for methadone/thorazine/valium/prozac/etc. exempts the user from sanctions. During the three years that I worked at the agency, I administered many drug tests. Through some fortuitous circumstance – perhaps that the element of surprise was intentionally unsuccessful – none of the patients ever tested positive, and nothing I did was ever responsible for sending anyone to prison.

That was over a decade ago, but it is only now that I fully understand the medical profession's abhorrence at self-medication. I received my holistic health training under the umbrella of the ancient teaching of Indian philosophy. Self-regulation and assuming full responsibility for one's own ailments is actually the goal of life in all ancient religio-philosophy. Yet, it is the antithesis of the Western Medical Model which fosters complete dependence on the almighty doctor (and the pharmaceutical/insurance industry). Obviously, anything that smacks of autonomous wisdom threatens the power of the state. If we get permission by the doctor, pay the pharmacist, or even obtain our numbness at the hands of the bartender who collects the government's taxes – if we change our brain waves with sugar, deaden them with TV – still we are not expanded in consciousness, and the threat of true sight does not loom. Only the psychedelics can terrorize the powers that be, for with them we are able to rebalance our psyches and neutralize our dis-ease – and we can grow them, forage for them and pay no government taxes (or insurance premiums). To self-medicate ourselves, to be autonomous, to make choices, to grow in wisdom and not in status – this will eventually topple the establishment – and they know it.

A Letter From Jail

Joan Bello, POW

Dear Friends & Holy Smokers: It looks curiously like any sleep-away camp, but without clue as to the season, year or even the country. It's 2 AM, and the overhead fixtures have been turned off for the past 3 hours. Everyone is asleep in their bunks but me.

Unusually bright night lights cast an eerie yellow outline of 22 single beds around the perimeter of a conspicuously barren room. There are no decorations on the walls, no night stands, no curtains on the eight plastic windows that obviously never open, and no clock. A few beds have pictures taped to headboards showing children and memories from different times.

The camp fantasy has quickly faded to the sinister reality. If I unhitch my usual thinking process – and let the emanation of this unnatural conglomerate of women impinge on my consciousness – I can actually feel an overwhelming and grossly inappropriate emotion of sheer indifference.

They say human beings will adjust to nearly any situation, accepting even the most uncomfortable conditions. The women here have surely done just that. They live in limbo, wondering when their time to rejoin life on the outside will come. Most of them are without financial resources, which automatically relegates them to sitting in jail – often for nearly a year – even though they have never been convicted of anything.

Once incarcerated, the injustice and inhumanity of the system becomes obvious. Sanity is maintained by an assumed apathy and quiet resignation. But I am acutely aware that this outward display of acceptance is just a defense mechanism against the rage that seethes in other women inmates – as I feel it too.

I understand for the first time what an unjust and cruel society we have conceived and why so many deprived people are driven to violence. I can taste the fear of having no freedom. I feel the fury of an unfamiliar anger which leads to images of revenge. But, miraculously, I am also experiencing all this from a distance.

I am in the meditative zone of being high. Here in jail, alone and remembering the sacred effect of the Marijuana Spirit, I am one with that vibration. I am in awe of the realization that over years and years of experience with being high by the grace of Holy Hemp that I have learned how to uncouple from the conditioning without benefit of the embodied *sativa*. The Grace of the Spirit within the cannabis plant has been imparted to me just by mentation!

Ironically, the magnificence of this hallowed experience is the reason why I am in jail, and why my husband sat in jail before me, not to mention the hundreds of thousands of peace-loving Americans who are presently incarcerated. Those of us who are the casualties in the front lines of the marijuana witch hunt are, of course, the best versed in all the depraved reasons our militaristic government is waging this criminal war on innocent citizens. Our numbers sadly keep growing as our commitment to the inalienable, natural right to medicate ourselves, pursue our own methods toward enjoyment, and worship the Divinity in the best way we can imagine grows ever stronger, gathering more and more people from all walks of life and all disciplines of science. Our prisons are inadequate to house what has become the most populated prison-society in the developed world because our laws define natural actions as crimes. The political system that upholds this foolhardy, cruel, unjustifiable policy is bolstered by the drive for profit.

The prison industry is booming, the police-state tactics are escalating, lawyers and judges are inundated with work as our inner cities are starving, our corporate giants are downsizing to maintain their profit margins, the medical profession is closing ranks around the pharmaceutical synthetics even as the death toll in side effects reaches horrendous proportions – all while one natural plant could ease the pain and suffering of so many sick and dying people, help save our dangerously diminishing forests from further exploitation, feed the billions of hungry, unfortunate people around the globe, and cleanse the toxins from the air we breath – and certainly increase the breathing capacity of us all.

I spoke to Michael Keleinman of Capital City Distributors in Austin who ordered some of my books the other day. He gave me what I think is the best way to sign off in these times of intolerance and injustice: "Never Give Up!"

Interesting Facts

"True, the Founding Fathers had provided for a specific right to bear arms, but the only reason they'd nothing to say about the right to plant seeds (was).because it never would have occurred to them that any state might care to abridge that right. After all, they were writing on hemp paper." Michael Pollan, quoting California flower grower, Will Fulton Harper's Magazine, April 1997.

"The smoking of cannabis, even long term, is not harmful to health." (Editorial, "Deglamorising cannabis," The Lancet, Vol. 346, No. 8985, November 11, 1995, p.1241)

Apparently, in Amsterdam where use of illicit drugs is made possible due to the hassle free (illicit) availability of that type of drug, the use of cannabis satisfies almost all curiosity. Small numbers of experienced cannabis users try other illicit substances, mostly cocaine and ecstasy. *"Cannabis Use, A Stepping Stone to Other Drugs?"* The Case of Amsterdam, by Peter Cohen and Arjan Sas.

"Perhaps the most pointed statement Wednesday to the powers of pot came from Keith Vines, a prosecutor in the San Francisco district attorney's office. In 1990, Vines prosecuted what was one of the biggest drug busts in the city's history. Three years later, he was near death because of AIDS wasting syndrome. The recom-mendation: marijuana. 'As a patient, I made the decision to save my life,' said Vines, a plaintiff in the case who still uses marijuana for medical purposes." From Los Angeles Times, May 1, 1997 (Copyright Los Angeles Times)

Washington, August 8, (Reuter) - Evidence shows that smoking marijuana can have healthy effects and further studies should be made into its medical value, according to a report to the U.S. National Institutes of Health released on Friday.

D.P. Tashkin: Marijuana Smoking and Lung Function, April 3, 1997
"No difference in lung function for heavy marijuana smokers and nonsmokers".